Structured Exercises in

WELLNESS
Promotion

Volume

4

Structured Exercises in

WELLNESS

Promotion

**A Handbook for
Trainers, Educators, Group Leaders**

Volume

4

**Edited by
Nancy Loving Tubesing, EdD
Donald A Tubesing, MDiv, PhD**

REPRODUCTION POLICY

Unless otherwise noted, your purchase of this volume entitles you to reproduce a modest quantity of the worksheets that appear in this book for your education/training activities. For this limited worksheet reproduction no special additional permission is needed. However the following statement, in total, must appear on all copies that you reproduce.

> Reproduced from *Structured Exercises in Wellness Promotion, Volume 4*, Nancy Loving Tubesing and Donald A. Tubesing, Editors. © 1994 Whole Person Associates, 210 W Michigan, Duluth, MN 55802.

Specific prior written permission is required from the publisher for any reproduction of a complete or adapted exercise with trainer instructions, or large-scale reproduction of worksheets, or for inclusion of material in another publication. Licensing or royalty arrangement requests for this usage must be submitted in writing and approved prior to any such use.

For further information please write for our Permissions Guidelines and Standard Permissions Form. Permission requests must be submitted at least 30 days in advance of your scheduled printing or reproduction.

Library of Congress Cataloging in Publication Data

Structured exercises in wellness promotion : A handbook for trainers, educators, and
 group leaders / Nancy Loving Tubesing and Donald A. Tubesing, eds.
 192p. 23cm.
   Summary: A collection of thirty-six exercises for wellness promotion to be used
 by trainers and facilitators in group settings.
   ISBN 1-57025-021-9 (v.4 : pbk) : $29.95
     1. Health-Education, problems, exercises, etc. 2. Health—education and
 problems. I. Title. II. Tubesing, Nancy Loving III. Tubesing, Donald A.
 RA440.5.S77   1988, 1994
 613'.2—dc19   83-61074

Printed in the United States of America

10 9 8 7 6 5 4 3 2 1

Published by:

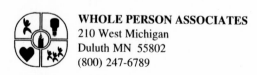

WHOLE PERSON ASSOCIATES
210 West Michigan
Duluth MN 55802
(800) 247-6789

PREFACE

*Over a decade ago we launched an experiment in health education—the Whole Person series of **Structured Exercises in Wellness Promotion** and **Structured Exercises in Stress Management**. We believed that it was time to move beyond peptalks and handouts to an experiential approach that actively involves the participant—as a whole person—in the learning process.*

*What began as an experiment has become a catalyst for dramatic changes in health promotion and education!**Structured Exercises** volumes have found their way into the libraries of trainers, consultants, group workers, and health professionals around the world. We're proud that these volumes have become classics—the resource of choice for planning stress management and wellness promotion programs.*

Our purpose in publishing this series was to foster inter-professional networking and to provide a framework though which we can all share our most effective ideas with each other. As you will soon discover, we scoured the country looking for the most innovative, effective teaching designs used by the most creative consultants and trainers in business, health care and social services, then included some of their most imaginative ideas in this volume.

Many of the exercises we designed ourselves and refined in hundreds of workshops we've conducted over the past twenty years. Some are new combinations of time-tested group process activities. Others were submitted by people like you who continually strive to add the creative touch to their teaching.

*The layout of **Structured Exercises** is designed for easy photocopying of worksheets, handouts and preparation notes. Please take advantage of our generous policy for reproduction—but also please be fair to the creative individuals who have so generously shared their ideas with you.*

☞ *You may duplicate worksheets and handouts for use in training or educational events—as long as you use the proper citation as indicated on the copyright page. Please also give written credit to the original contributor. Whenever we've been able to track down the source of an idea, we've noted it. Please do the same when you share these ideas with others.*

☞ *However, all materials in this volume are still protected by copyright. Prior written permission from Whole Person Press is required if you plan large scale reproduction or distribution of any portion of this book. If you wish to include any material or adaptation in another publication, you must have permission in writing before proceeding. Please send us your request and proposal at least thirty days in advance.*

Structured Exercises *are now available in two convenient formats. This small-format softcover version is produced with a new book binding process that stays open on your desk or podium for easy reference, and lies flat on the photocopier for quick duplication of worksheets.*

Many trainers enjoy the wide margins and larger type of the full-size looseleaf format, which provides plenty of space for you to add your own workshop designs, examples, chalktalk notes, and process reminders for your presentations. The looseleaf version also includes a complete package of camera-ready worksheet masters for easy reproduction of professional-looking handouts.

☞ *See page 156 in the Resources section for complete descriptions and ordering information for worksheet masters and companion volumes of the* **Stress** *and* **Wellness** *series in softcover and looseleaf formats.*

We are grateful to the many creative trainers who have so generously shared their "best" with you in this volume (see page 149) as well as others in the series. We hope that the ideas here stimulate your own creative juices.

So, go ahead. Strive to bring your teaching alive in new ways. Expand your stress management approach. Continue to touch and motivate people with learning experiences that engage and challenge them as whole persons.

Then let us know what works well for you. We'd love to consider your new ideas for inclusion in a future volume so that we can carry on the tradition of providing this international exchange of innovative teaching designs.

Duluth MN   *Nancy Loving Tubesing*
January 1994   *Donald A Tubesing*

INTRODUCTION

Wellness is the hot topic of the decade. If you're prepared to address the issue, you'll get plenty of opportunities. If you creatively involve people in the learning process, reflecting assessing, prioritizing, sorting, planning for change and affirming progress, your teaching will be much more helpful than even the most entertaining lecture.

Structured Exercises in Wellness Promotion, Volume 4 provides 36 designs you can use for getting people involved, whatever the setting and time constraints, whatever the sophistication of the audience. To aid you in the selection of appropriate content and process to meet your objectives, the exercises are grouped into five broad categories:

> *Icebreakers:* These short (10–20 minutes) exercises are designed to introduce people to each other and to open up participants' thinking process regarding wellness. They are lively! Each engages people actively in the topic and with each other. Try combining an icebreaker with an exercise from the wellness or self-care section for an instant evening progam.

> *Wellness Exploration:* These exercises explore the issue of wellness from the whole person perspective. Rather than focus merely on the physical, these processes help people examine their lifestyle. You'll find a mixture of moderate-length assessments (30–60 minutes) and major theme developers (60–90 minutes). Any exercise can easily be contracted or expanded to fit your purpose.

> *Self-Care Strategies:* These exercises promote personal responsibility for well-being. Participants examine their self-care patterns and explore specific self-care strategies in different life dimensions: physical (diet, relaxation, fitness), mental, rational, spiritual and lifestyle well-being. (10–60 minutes)

> *Action Planning/Closure:* These exercises help participants draw together their insights and determine the actions they wish to take on their own behalf. (20–40 minutes)

> *Energizers:* The energizers are designed to perk up the group whenever fatigue sets in. Sprinkle them throughout your program to illustrate skills or concepts. Try one for a change of pace—everyone's juices (including yours!) will be flowing again in 5–10 minutes.

The format is designed for easy use. You'll find that each exercise is described completely, including: goals, group size, time frame, materials needed, step-by-step process instructions, and variations.

☞ *Special instructions for the trainer and scripts to be read to the group are typed in italics.*

✔ Questions to ask the group are preceded by a check.

➤ Directions for group activities are indicated by an arrow.

● Mini-lecture notes are preceded by a bullet.

Although the processes are primarily described for large group (25 to 100 people) workshop settings, most of the exercises work just as well with small groups, and many are appropriate for individual therapy or personal reflection.

If you are teaching in the workshop or large group setting, we believe that the use of small discussion groups is the most potent learning structure available to you. We've found that groups of four persons each provide ample air time and a good variety of interaction. If possible, let groups meet together two or three different times during the learning experience before forming new groups.

These personal sharing groups allow people to make positive contact with each other and encourage them to personalize their experience in depth. On evaluations, some people will say "Drop this," others will say, "Give us more small group time," but most will report that the time you give them to share with each other becomes the heart of the workshop.

If you are working with an intact group of 12 people or less, you may want to keep the whole group together for process and discussion time rather than divide into the suggested four or six person groups.

Each trainer has personal strengths, biases, pet concepts and processes. We expect and encourage you to expand and modify what you find here to accommodate your style. Adjust the exercises as you see fit. Bring these designs to life for your participants by inserting your own content and examples into your teaching. Experiment!

And when you come up with something new, let us know . . .

CONTENTS

ICEBREAKERS

WELLNESS EXPLORATION

SELF-CARE STRATEGIES

PLANNING & CLOSURE

GROUP ENERGIZERS

RESOURCES

Icebreakers

109 INTRODUCTIONS 7

In these three quick introductions, participants find a fruit that fits (**An Apple a Day**), identify their personality type (**Hippocratic Humors**) and use a familiar material in a new way to tell their stories (**TP Tales**).

GOALS

To elicit participation from everyone.

To get acquainted.

GROUP SIZE

Unlimited; with more than 15 participants, divide into smaller groups (6–12 people) for introductions.

TIME FRAME

10–15 minutes; allow more time for larger groups.

MATERIALS NEEDED

An Apple a Day: Selection of fresh apples, one for each participant. **Hippocratic Humors**: Blackboard or newsprint easel. **TP Tales**: One roll of toilet paper for each small group of participants.

Introduction A: AN APPLE A DAY

1) The trainer directs participants to form groups of eight.

   ☞ *With 16–20 people, divide into odd and even birth-date groups. In a very large group, you may want to use a pairs–quartets–octets process to form groups. Don't worry about the exact numbers. Just make sure there are about the same number in each group and that the proper number of apples get distributed.*

2) The trainer distributes a sack of apples to each group and gives instructions for introductions.

   ➤ Pile the apples in the center of your group so that everyone can look at them.

   ➤ Each person should pick an apple that reminds you of yourself in some way.

➤ Once you've found the apple of your eye, study it closely for one minute and notice all the ways that it is like you.

➤ I'll tell you when the time is up.

3) The trainer allows about 2 minutes for the choosing and studying process, then interrupts with further instructions for introductions.

➤ Polish your apple a little bit and put it back in the middle of the circle. Someone should volunteer to mix them up.

➤ Now each person should find your own apple again and use it to introduce yourself to the others by telling:

➢ Some area of your life that shines (eg, "I walk 5 miles a day," or "I really love my job and find it stimulating");

➢ One blemish you've learned to live with (eg, "I have a reading disability," or "I have a trick knee that buckles without warning").

4) Participants take turns introducing themselves.

Introduction B: HIPPOCRATIC HUMORS

1) The trainer briefly introduces the Hippocratic concept of "body humors."

● Hippocrates, the ancient Greek physician recognized as the father of medicine, believed that disease results from an imbalance of the four body humors: sanguine, choleric, melancholic and phlegmatic.

● Modern medicine has replaced Hippocrates' theory of humors with a more sophisticated explanation of disease processes, but we are beginning to rediscover the value of his exhortation that medicine should build the patient's strength through diet and hygiene, resorting to other treatment only when absolutely necessary.

2) The trainer describes some typical qualities that could be associated with each of the four Hippocratic humors, writing the characteristics on the blackboard or newsprint.

● **SANGUINE**: warm, friendly, outgoing, optimistic.

● **CHOLERIC**: strong, self-willed, driven, organized.

● **MELANCHOLIC**: imaginative, creative, sensitive, artistic.

● **PHLEGMATIC**: steady, easy-going, likable, dependable.

3) The trainer instructs participants to select the body humor that best fits their temperament these days and introduce themselves to the group.

Introduction C: TP TALES

1) The trainer passes a roll of toilet paper around each group, instructing participants to tear off as much as they might need to blow their nose.

2) After everyone has taken a portion, participants are invited to introduce themselves one-by-one, telling one interesting fact about themselves for each square of toilet paper.

   ☞ *You might want to close on a humorous note (eg, "Now, if you still need to blow your nose, go ahead!").*

VARIATION

■ Participants save one or more squares of TP to use in a second round. After the introductions in *Step 2* people use the remaining squares to name their expectations for the learning experience.

TRAINER'S NOTES

An Apple a Day submitted by Lyman Coleman. TP Tales is adapted from an idea in Group Magazine by Mary Albert.

110 LOST AND FOUND

In this thought-provoking icebreaker, participants describe health-related gains and losses they have experienced.

GOALS

To review personal wellness attitudes and behaviors.

To get acquainted.

GROUP SIZE

Unlimited.

TIME FRAME

10–15 minutes

MATERIALS NEEDED

Blank paper for everyone.

PROCESS

1) The trainer introduces the exercise with a quick overview of wellness concepts, highlighting the growing awareness among health care providers that our attitudes and personal choices have a profound effect on our total well-being.

2) The trainer invites participants to reflect over the past year and consider which of their health-related attitudes and behaviors have changed in that time. To help people get focused she invites them to note their responses as she asks the questions below.

    ☞ *To maximize the effectiveness of this reflection process, be sure to give lots of examples tailored to the background of the audience and the objectives of your learning experience. Encourage people to recall both positive and negative changes.*

    ➤ During the past year, what health-related habits or behaviors have you cut down, given up or lost (eg, reduced "spare tire," quit smoking, ate less red meat, stopped taking tranquilizers, lost my time for play, swore off caffeine)?

    ➤ What about *attitudes, beliefs* or *myths?* Have you discarded, given up or lost any during the past year (eg, gave up believing I have to be a size 10, stopped hating vegetables, lost my sense of wonder, quit pretending I get enough exercise, etc)?

➤ Now, think about *health-related behaviors* you've *found* during the past year. What new habits have you acquired? What new behaviors have you taken on (eg, started walking program, buckle my seatbelt, floss my teeth, do a monthly breast self-exam, take time for daily meditation/relaxation, etc)?

➤ What *new notions about health* have you discovered this year? Have you *found* any new or renewed motivations, resolutions, convictions, attitudes (eg, I believe my headaches are related to stress; I'm convinced alcohol is harmful to health; although I'm not a jock, I can exercise, I have ultimate responsibility for my own health, etc)?

3) Participants take turns introducing themselves by briefly sharing something they have *lost* and something they have *found* during the past year (1 minute each).

☞ *With more than 15 people, divide into smaller groups (6–10 persons each) for these introductions.*

4) The trainer asks the group to comment on the general themes expressed by participants and uses these insights to provide transition to the next content segment.

TRAINER'S NOTES

111 HEARTS AT RISK

Serious and humorous brainstorming in small groups provides a good warm-up to an in-depth presentation on risk factors for cardiovascular disease.

GOALS

To increase awareness of factors that affect the risk of heart attack and coronary heart disease.

To promote small group interaction and bonding.

GROUP SIZE

Unlimited.

TIME FRAME

10–15 minutes

MATERIALS NEEDED

Blackboard or newsprint.

PROCESS

1) The trainer defines a *risk factor* for heart disease:
   - A *risk factor* is an attribute you have, or to which you are exposed, that increases the likelihood that you will develop some form of coronary heart disease.

2) The trainer instructs participants to write down three qualities or behaviors they believe could be risk factors for heart disease.

   ☞ *Reassure participants that it's fine if they are not sure—that's a great reason for coming to a presentation like this! Do encourage people to take a guess. Or suggest that they think of someone they know who had a heart attack. What did everyone say that the person "did wrong" or "should have done?"*

3) Participants are instructed to pair up with someone they don't know, introduce themselves and tell each other the three risk factors they wrote down in *Step 2*. (1–2 minutes)

☞ *Participants might be embarrassed if they couldn't think of the "right" risk factors in Step 2. Tell them that there are many surprising risk factors. One of their "wild guesses" just might be right.*

4) The trainer gives instructions for the next round of introductions.

➤ Each pair find another pair and join to make a group of four.

➤ Go around the group. Introduce your partner to the others and mention what she said were the major risk factors.

5) The trainer interrupts after 2–3 minutes and instructs groups to decide on the ***three most likely risk factors*** from those posed by the group. When most groups have decided, he poses one further challenge:

➤ Go around the circle and be silly or creative in response to this question: *"What is almost certainly not a risk factor for heart disease?"*

☞ *Give a few off-beat examples (eg, shoe size, sign of the zodiac, left/right-handed, color of hair, etc).*

➤ After everyone has suggested a far-fetched possibility, decide together which is the most unlikely risk factor.

6) The trainer calls for reports from the group. He writes down each group's *three most likely risk factors* in one column, the *unlikely factors* in another column. He then uses the data generated to introduce a more detailed presentation on one or more of the documented major risk factors for heart disease: cigarette smoking, poor nutrition, poor exercise patterns, blood cholesterol levels, high blood pressure, diabetes. Other potential risk factors such as heredity, acute and chronic stress, obesity and alcohol abuse may also be covered.

☞ *For fun, try to find some relationship between the "absurd" risk factors and those that are documented by research. Stretch your imagination—or ask for assistance from the group.*

VARIATION

■ This exercise makes an excellent introduction to the *Health and Lifestyle* film and exercise (p 33) which covers risk factors and health-enhancing lifestyle changes in more detail.

Submitted by Donald B Ardell.

112 MAGIC DOOR

In this guided group fantasy, participants use the "magic" of visualization to prepare themselves for the learning experience.

GOALS

To create an atmosphere of expectancy for learning.

To explore the power of visualization as a creative model for approaching problems.

GROUP SIZE

Unlimited; also effective with individuals.

TIME FRAME

10–15 minutes

MATERIALS NEEDED

Magic Door guided fantasy script.

PROCESS

1) The trainer invites participants to join in an unusual warm-up that will help them remove themselves from the hectic here-and-now and prepare for adventure.

2) Participants are instructed to find a comfortable position with feet on the floor and eyes closed. The trainer asks them to relax, take a deep breath, and turn their attention inward.

3) The trainer reads the **Magic Door** script.

   ☞ *Read the script slowly, pausing frequently. Allow participants plenty of time to visualize each image and movement. Keep your voice low and soothing.*

4) Without breaking the mystical mood of the fantasy, the trainer uses images from the visualization to make a transition to the next activity (eg, "The beginning of a workshop is something like the hidden magic door . . . we're never sure exactly what we'll discover, but our curiosity draws us on . . . and there's usually an adventure in the process. Let's get started!").

MAGIC DOOR GUIDED FANTASY Script

As we begin, take another deep breath
and slowly bring your awareness into your feet . . . .
Now let your awareness rise up your lower legs . . .
into your knees . . . up into your thighs . . . your pelvis . . .
stomach . . . chest . . . shoulders . . .
down into your arms . . . hands. . . fingers . . .
up into your neck . . . and head . . . .
Allow your face to relax and concentrate on your breathing . . . .

Breathe slowly and softly . . . like a child sleeping . . . .
As you breathe . . . take yourself back to your childhood . . .
to a time when you were going to sleep and everything felt good . . . .
It is a very peaceful evening . . .
the stars are shining and you are cozily tucked into bed . . . .

Although you are almost asleep, your curiosity is awake
and you begin to wonder about the closet in your room . . . .
Somehow you know there is a magical door
hidden in the back of the closet . . . .
You get out of bed to investigate . . . and there it is . . .
hidden behind a curtain at the back . . . .

You pull back the curtain . . . open the hidden door . . .
and with a great sense of adventure,
enter the semi-darkness on the other side . . . .
There is a dim light to guide you as you begin to walk down a long spiral
staircase . . .
winding down, down, down . . . .
As you descend, your curiosity grows and grows.
You continue going down . . . slowly . . .
taking your time . . . and being careful to keep your balance . . . .

Finally you come to the bottom . . .
which opens into a large cavern filled with water . . . .
At the edge of the water is a boat . . .
tied to the base of the steps you have just climbed down . . . .
You enter the boat, untying it and releasing it from its dock . . . .

You lie down in the bottom of the boat
and wrap yourself in a comfortable blanket . . . .
The boat begins drifting with a natural current
that carries it across the waters of the cavern . . . .

©1994 Whole Person Press 210 W Michigan Duluth MN 55802   (800) 247-6789

Its natural rocking movement is very relaxing . . . .
The water laps gently against your boat with a soothing rhythm . . . .

At the other side of the cavern
your boat enters a large and long tunnel . . . .
The current moves more quickly now,
taking you far into the depths of the tunnel . . .
until off in the distance you see a light . . . .
The light grows as you move more quickly toward the end of the tunnel . . .
and at last you emerge into full daylight . . . .

You find yourself in a beautiful sunlit world . . .
with lovely rolling hills . . .
bright green and full of flowers, birds and flourishing nature . . . .
You can smell the fragrances of the different flowers
and hear the birds singing and the bees buzzing
as on a warm summer day . . . .

Your boat is now drifting toward the shore . . .
and gently lands so that you can easily get up
and explore the new world before you . . . .
You walk slowly up a hill to a large tree at the top . . . .
You sit down under the tree . . .
and looking around at this wonderful new land . . .
you prepare yourself for great adventure . . . .

When you are ready to begin . . . gently open your eyes . . . .

Submitted by Neil Young.

113 WHEEL OF FORTUNE

This fast-paced icebreaker gives participants an opportunity to discuss wellness attitudes with a succession of group members as they follow the "wheel of fortune's" spin.

GOALS

To consider attitudes and experiences related to wellness.

To promote self-disclosure and interaction among participants.

GROUP SIZE

Unlimited, as long as there is plenty of open space to make the "wheel of fortune."

TIME FRAME

10–15 minutes

MATERIALS NEEDED

Conversation Starters handout.

PROCESS

1) The trainer asks participants to pair up with a neighbor for introductions.

   ➤ Briefly tell each other about a favorite book or story from childhood. (2 minutes)

2) The trainer instructs the partners to decide who will be the *poker chip* and who will be the *silver dollar.*

3) The trainer gives instructions for making the *Wheel of Fortune.*

   ☞ *As participants move around the room, distribute the Conversation Starters handouts to everyone.*

   ➤ *Silver dollars* should form a circle in the middle of the room, with your backs to each other.

   ➤ *Poker chips* should stand facing your partners, forming a second, larger circle, facing inward.

4) As soon as the circle is formed, the trainer instructs participants to change partners for a new conversation.

➤ Poker chips should move one person to the left, so that everyone is facing a new partner.

5) The trainer calls the number of a **Conversation Starter** from the list and announces the format.

☞ *Choose Conversation Starters that apply to the theme of the session. Feel free to add humorous or serious ideas that are pertinent to your audience.*

➤ Each member of the pair has 30 seconds to respond to the sentence stem and elaborate briefly.

➤ *Silver dollars* begin.

6) After one minute, the trainer interrupts and instructs *poker chips* to move one person to the left again, and calls the number of another **Conversation Starter**. Each partner has 30 seconds to respond.

7) *Step 6* is repeated several times, until the group is warmed up to the subject and each other.

VARIATION

■ This process is also effective with small groups. Instead of dividing into pairs, the trainer divides members into groups of 4–8 people. When the trainer calls a number, group members take turns responding to the Conversation Starter. The trainer should allow several members to respond to a given Conversation Starter before calling another number. When the trainer calls another number, the next group member responds to the new Conversation Starter. Continue this process at a rapid pace until your time is up, or until the energy of the group begins to fall.

CONVERSATION STARTERS

1. My favorite childhood story or book was . . . .
2. When I get a cold, I . . .
3. If I could give up one bad habit . . . .
4. When I'm angry . . . .
5. My doctor . . . .
6. To take better care of myself I should . . . .
7. The part of my body where I collect tension . . . .
8. Happiness is . . . .
9. The worst thing in life is . . . .
10. One thing I have difficulty accepting about myself . . . .
11. Health is . . . .
12. The best measure of health . . . .
13. If I could change one thing in the environment I would . . . .
14. I'm killing myself in slow stages by . . . .
15. My life is full of . . .
16. My experience with aerobic exercise . . . .
17. If I changed jobs . . . .
18. When it comes to health, I feel responsible for . . .
19. Healthy foods . . . .
20. When I feel sad . . . .
21. The best dietary change I could make . . . .
22. When I'm excited . . . .
23. When I get sick . . . .
24. The most important thing I can do to improve my health . . . .
25. I like to spend my leisure time . . . .
26. Wellness is . . . .
27. Illness is . . . .
28. My highest aspiration . . . .
29. The most important thing in my life . . . .
30. I look forward to . . . .
31. My favorite cartoon or comic strip is . . . .
32. Love is . . . .
33. My physical activity is . . . .
34. The best thing in life is . . . .
35. Life . . . .
36. If my body could speak . . . .
37. Don't tease me about . . . .
38. Five years from now . . . .
39. When everything looks hopeless . . . .
40. Exercise . . .
41. I'm critical of myself . . . .
42. When I'm under stress . . . .
43. When I feel worried . . . .
44. I like to be touched . . . .
45. I believe . . . .
46. The worst way to die . . . .
47. The best way to die . . . .
48. With 6 months to live, I . . . .

©1994 Whole Person Press 210 W Michigan Duluth MN 55802   (800) 247-6789

114 WELLNESS EMBLEM

Participants "picture" wellness by creating a wellness emblem symbolizing their values, goals and achievements.

GOALS

To stimulate reflection on topics to be considered during the session.

To articulate goals for the learning experience.

To get acquainted with several other participants.

GROUP SIZE

Unlimited.

TIME FRAME

15–20 minutes

MATERIALS NEEDED

Wellness Emblem worksheets.

PROCESS

1) The trainer distributes **Wellness Emblem** worksheets and announces
   that participants are going to create a wellness emblem that depicts their
   values, goals and achievements.

2) The trainer gives instructions for completing the diagram.

   ➤ Choose one of the two shapes to represent yourself.

   ➤ I am going to ask you a series of questions. Use a different compartment of the emblem to respond to each one. You may use words or
   pictures in your response.

   ☞ *Pose the questions one at a time, with examples. Pause for
   about a minute between each one so participants can fill in
   that portion of the emblem.*

   *If participants ask how they'll know when to use the center
   portion of the daisy emblem, tell them to fill it in whenever they
   come to a response that is particularly significant to them.*

   ➤ Name a *personal health issue* that deeply concerns you (eg, heart
   disease, overweight, smoking, etc). Draw or write your response in
   one compartment of the emblem.

> What *self-care routine or habit* do you practice that you're particularly proud of (eg, relaxation routines, physical exercise, flossing teeth, etc)?

> What are *three words* that you consider essential to wellness?

> What's *something you've achieved* over the past year that means a lot to you (eg, building a deck, job promotion, computer literacy, etc)? Remember, you can write or draw a symbol to represent your achievement.

> What is one of your *core values* (eg, self-fulfillment, honesty, independence, etc)?

> Finally, in the last compartment, represent your *goal or wish for this course/session/workshop.*

3) The trainer instructs participants to pair up with a neighbor (preferably someone they don't know well). As soon as everyone has a partner, she gives instructions for the introductions.

> Introduce yourselves.

> Then take one minute each to describe in detail the self-care routine you put into your emblem. Describe this habit in detail; try to "sell" the routine to your partner.

>> Why did you start doing it in the first place?

>> How long have you been doing it?

> Why do you keep doing it? What keeps you motivated?

4) The trainer directs pairs to join with another pair, making quartets. Participants are instructed to introduce themselves, then to share with each other the three essential words of wellness from their emblems.

5) After 2–3 minutes the trainer interrupts and instructs participants to make groups of eight (two quartets) for another round of introductions. Participants introduce themselves, then share the contents of any remaining compartment of the emblem and talk about their wishes or goals for the course. (5–8 minutes)

6) The trainer reconvenes the entire group and asks for examples of *wellness words* or *health issues of concern* that participants put in the other compartments. She then uses one or more of these contributions as a bridge to the next agenda item.

WELLNESS EMBLEM

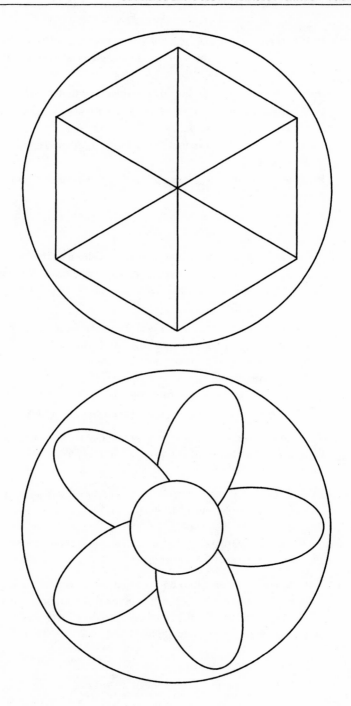

Wellness
Exploration

115 WELLNESS PROFILE

In this assessment, participants create a "wellness profile" that plots their own measure of where they are now and what changes they would like to make.

GOALS

To recognize personal wellness patterns.

To plan how to improve key areas of well-being.

GROUP SIZE

Unlimited.

TIME FRAME

15–20 minutes

MATERIALS NEEDED

A **Wellness Profile** worksheet for each participant.

PROCESS

1) The trainer begins with a brief chalktalk on wellness concepts, emphasizing the following points:

- **Wellness is a philosophy of wholeness**, the appreciation that everything you do, think, feel and believe has an impact on your state of health. In order to be truly well, we need to attend to and nurture body, mind and spirit.

- **We can view health/illness as a continuum** that stretches from disease on one extreme to high-level wellness on the other. If we settle for the neutral midpoint, "not being sick," we may miss out on the vitality, energy and self-actualization that is our potential.

- **Wellness is a choice**. We are always growing and changing in our awareness and actions. We place ourselves on the continuum and decide which way to go. No matter what your current state of health, you can move toward more positive health.

2) The trainer passes out **Wellness Profile** worksheets and explains that the self-assessment *Profile* will give participants a "snapshot" of how they are doing in eight key areas of well-being.

3) The trainer guides the group through the worksheet, reading the following descriptions.

> ☞ *Pause for about 30 seconds after each item to allow time for participants to consider and mark their response.*

➤ **Overall energy level**. Over the past week, did you feel as if you had sufficient energy to do what you wanted to do? Did you have more or less energy than usual?

> ➣ Place an "X" on the line to indicate how you would rate the *energy level* area of your life during the past week—fair, good, great or somewhere in between. Then jot down some examples of what influenced your placement of the X.

➤ **Nutritional awareness.** How did you feel about the nutritional choices you made last week? Did you feel that you had enough knowledge to make the right choices?

> ➣ Mark your assessment of *nutritional awareness* for the past week and note examples.

➤ **Physical activity**. Were you satisfied with the amount of exercise you got last week? Were you more or less active than usual?

> ➣ Put an X on the line to represent your *activity level* and give examples.

➤ **Stress management**. Did you use any stress management techniques last week? Were they appropriate and constructive? Did you feel more stressed than usual? More stressed than you would like?

> ➣ Rate yourself on how well you *coped with stress* last week and mark it on your worksheet.

➤ **Contact with others**. This may describe either the time you are required to spend with others, or the time you are able to spend with others, depending on your perspective. Do you need more time alone? More time with other people? What about the quality of time you spent with others?

> ➣ Evaluate your *relationships* last week on the continuum.

➤ **Personally meaningful moments**. Did you engage in any activities this past week that provided meaning to you (eg, spending time with a special person, reading an inspiring book, making a contribution to society, etc)?

> ➣ Rank yourself on this *spiritual indicator* of well-being.

➤ **Quiet time**. Are you satisfied with the amount and quality of time you spent last week in spiritual pursuits and centering yourself? Do you feel inwardly peaceful?

    ➤ Record your assessment of *quiet time* on the worksheet.

➤ **Self-responsibility**. During the past week, did you take charge of your life? Did you make your own choices about your feelings and behaviors? Were you assertive when you needed to be? Are you pleased with your self-care pattern?

    ➤ Mark your X on this final *self-care* continuum.

4) The trainer invites participants to study their overall *Wellness Profile* for the past week, reflect on the following questions and record their insights.

➤ What relationships do you see among the different areas?

➤ Are there any surprises in your profile?

➤ What areas would you most like to change?

➤ At the bottom of the profile, complete the sentence, *"My wellness profile for the past week is . . ."*

5) The trainer asks participants to look at their Profile again, this time focusing on the week ahead.

➤ For each key area, decide where you'd like to be on that continuum *next week,* and *make a star* to mark your goal. Be optimistic, but realistic—you can't change everything in just a week. Of course, there may be some areas where you don't want to change.

    ☞ *You may want to guide the group through each area as in Step 3. This will remind people of the specific components and will help keep everyone together.*

6) The trainer invites participants to consider how they might reach their goals.

➤ Look over your Profile, comparing the **X's** (last week) with the **stars** (next week).

➤ For each area where you'd like to improve, think about specific steps you could take during the next week to improve in that area. These steps may be changes in behavior, attitude or environment.

➤ As a group we will be brainstorming possible strategies for improvement. During this process, write at least one positive step for each of your target areas in the *Movement* section at the bottom of the worksheet.

7) The trainer focuses on one area at a time, soliciting from the group ideas for positive change and adding examples of his own as necessary from the list below.

☞ *After several ideas are generated for an area by the group, remind those participants who are hoping to make changes in this area to write down an idea or two that might help them make that improvement. Then move on to the next assessment area.*

- **Overall Energy Level.** Drink less coffee; focus on positive thoughts instead of negative ones; get enough sleep.
- **Nutritional Awareness.** Rid my kitchen of junk food; read the labels on all prepared foods I buy at the supermarket; eat at least two servings of fresh fruit or vegetables a day.
- **Physical Activity.** Walk at least 10 minutes a day; go to the health club three times this week.
- **Stress Management.** Take a 10-minute relaxation break at some point every day; keep a diary of my physical, mental and emotional reactions to stress; learn and practice a new stress management technique.
- **Contact with Others.** Call an old friend; really talk to my family during dinner; accept only those invitations that I want to accept.
- **Personally Meaningful Moments.** Volunteer a few hours for a cause I believe in; read a good book; spend some time at a hobby I've been neglecting.
- **Quiet Time.** Attend a religious or other spiritual service; set aside a special time to think about where my life is going and what I want to do with it.
- **Self-responsibility.** Go an entire day without saying, "I don't care," "It's up to you," or "It's not my fault;" practice making decisions and answering questions without elaborate explanations, apologies or excuses.

8) The trainer summarizes the exercise, emphasizing the following points:
- The *Wellness Profile* is valuable because it provides an overall picture of how you're doing at a given time. Use the *Wellness Profile* for periodic assessment to see if you're remaining in balance.
- Wellness is a lifetime project, but changes take place weekly or even daily. The sum total of your *Wellness Profile* can be altered by the choices you make every day.

VARIATION

■ As part of *Step 7*, participants gather into small "consultation" groups to brainstorm ideas for positive change and to discuss their plans for improving their *Wellness Profiles*. The trainer may solicit examples from each group and write the suggestions on a blackboard or newsprint.

TRAINER'S NOTES

Adapted from the weekly wellness profile in Larry Tobin's intriguing calendar/ planner, Time Well Spent.

©1994 Whole Person Press 210 W Michigan Duluth MN 55802   (800) 247-6789

WELLNESS PROFILE

	FAIR	GOOD	GREAT	COMMENTS
Overall Energy Level				
Nutritional Awareness				
Physical Activity				
Stress Management				
Contact With Others				
Meaningful Moments				
Quiet Time				
Self-Responsibility				

My wellness profile for the past week is . . .

MOVEMENT

Over the next week, I will take the following steps:

Overall Energy Level:

Nutritional Awareness:

Physical Activity:

Stress Management:

Contact With Others:

Personally Meaningful Moments:

Quiet Time:

Self-Responsibility:

116 WHOLE PERSON POTPOURRI

Participants envision whole person well-being and develop innovative strategies for moving toward that vision in unusual settings. Small group *esprit de corps* and good-natured humor are energizing side benefits of this creative and entertaining process.

GOALS

To explore a variety of options for promoting whole person well-being.

To demonstrate the power of societal patterns.

To promote creativity and humor.

GROUP SIZE

This exercise works best with 40–100 people; with fewer than 40 participants, the energy and creativity may be diminished; the logistics are just too cumbersome with more than 100.

TIME FRAME

60–90 minutes

MATERIALS NEEDED

Whole Person Potpourri Creative Challenge cards (prepared in advance by the trainer) and designated supplies for each small group; newsprint, water color markers, masking tape.

☞ *It's best to determine in advance the number of small groups you will be working with. The exercise works best with 12 to 20 separate small groups of 4–8 people each (eg, with 50 people, plan for 12 four-person groups; with 100 people, try 13 eight-person groups or 16 six-person groups or 20 five-person groups, etc). If you're not sure how many participants to expect, prepare plenty of **Creative Challenge** cards and accompanying supplies and adjust the group composition at the last minute.*

PROCESS

☞ *Allow plenty of time before the session to prepare materials for participants and to set up the room.*

*Consult the **Potpourri** list on pp 28–32 and decide which activities you would like to try with your audience (a different one for each* *small group). Cut out the appropriate assignments (or write them on notecards) and collect the accessory items needed to accomplish the various tasks. You may want to use a paper bag for each group to hold the supplies and the instruction card.*

Each group will need a "headquarters" in the room. Hang sheets of newsprint (one per group) at equally spaced intervals, making sure that no furniture blocks access.

Be sure that you have plenty of water-color markers—permanent markers will bleed through the paper and onto the walls! Label the newsprint sheets in sequence, PHYSICAL, MENTAL, SPIRITUAL, RELATIONAL and EMOTIONAL, repeating the cycle until each sheet has a title.

Phase 1: Warm-Up (20–30 minutes)

1) The trainer introduces the exercise with a few remarks on wellness as a whole person issue and then divides participants into the predetermined number of small groups and directs them to find a "home base" at one of the newsprints.

   ☞ *This process can be chaotic. With a large group you may want to number off quickly (by 15's for 15 groups) and give a number to each newsprint. Each group should have its own water-based felt-tip marker.*

2) The trainer instructs each group to brainstorm creative, wellness-enhancing behaviors that correspond with the dimension of whole-person well-being listed on their newsprint (physical, mental, spiritual, etc) and gives guidelines for the process.

   ➤ The shortest person in the group should act as a recorder.

   ➤ As a group, brainstorm together creative, wellness-enhancing behaviors for your designated area of the whole person. List as many ideas as you can in the next two minutes.

   ➤ Write down every suggestion, even the most bizarre or offhand humorous comments. Don't censor anything. The more creative the better.

3) After 2–3 minutes the trainer calls time and directs the groups to move one newsprint sheet to their right, clockwise around the room. Groups are instructed to spend 1 minute reading what the previous group has written, then 2 minutes adding their own creative ideas for wellness-

enhancing behaviors applicable to the area of whole person well-being designated on this newsprint sheet.

☞ *Encourage groups to be as creative and zany as possible, hitch-hiking on ideas of the previous group and combining unusual elements and activities to increase the humor.*

4) The trainer repeats *Step 3* one or two more cycles, depending on the time available and the energy of the groups.

☞ *Keep encouraging participants to stretch their imaginations and be as "off the wall as possible" with the ideas they record.*

You may need to supply additional pieces of newsprint in some locations as they begin to fill up with ideas.

5) The trainer asks groups to rotate once more to the right. This time they are instructed to read through the contents of their newsprint(s) and select and circle the three most creative, humorous ideas recorded there. (3–4 minutes)

6) The trainer calls on each group recorder in turn to name the dimension of well-being and read the list of most creative wellness-enhancers selected by their group.

☞ *This process needs to move swiftly, and usually the recorder will need to shout to be heard. Keep the pace fast to build the energy level.*

Phase 2: Creative Challenge   (40–60 minutes)

7) The trainer announces that each small group will now tackle a creative challenge that applies this whole person view of wellness in an unusual way.

➤ Welcome to the whole person creative challenge! Each small group will independently produce a whole person presentation for the rest of the participants.

➤ Each group will receive a different and distinct creative challenge.

➤ You will have 25 minutes to accomplish the task assigned to you.

➤ Your final presentation must involve every member of your small group in some way.

➤ Send the tallest person in your group up to the front to receive your creative challenge.

☞ *Hand out the instructions for assignments plus the necessary props to the group representatives, then send them quickly back to their groups to get to work. Do not let groups compare their assignments.*

8) Small groups spend 25 minutes completing their assignment and preparing their presentation.

☞ *Some people may need assurance that this is a serious task. You need to state clearly that in 25 minutes sharp they will make their whole person presentation to the rest of the participants.*

After 15 minutes, remind participants that they have only 10 minutes until "showtime." Encourage them to rehearse their presentation so that they are really ready. Remind groups that everyone must participate in the presentation.

9) After the groups have had 25 minutes for preparation, the trainer reconvenes the participants and announces that the presentations will begin. The trainer gives guidelines for the process:

➤ Before you begin your presentation, read your creative challenge out loud to the rest of us.

➤ All presentations are to be made from the front of the room and must include all the members of your small group.

➤ Listen and learn from the ideas that other groups share.

☞ *The performances will provide maximum humor, energy and insight if the pace moves rapidly. Don't let it drag. Politely thank each group following their presentation and immediately move on to the next. Be sure to hand the microphone to each group so that they can be heard well.*

10) After all presentations are completed, the trainer invites participants to give themselves a hand.

11) In closing, the trainer asks for comments, observations and insights on the multiple dimensions of whole person well-being.

VARIATIONS

■ The presentations may be treated as a contest. Appoint a panel of judges prior to the performances and call on them afterwards to announce awards for humor or merit that seem to fit.

■ This activity usually generates an amazing creative flow. The trainer may wish to collect all presentations, type them out, duplicate them and distribute the compilation to participants as a memento of the occasion.

■ This exercise can be preceded by an in-depth discussion of whole person well-being. The *Potpourri* then serves to enhance creativity and expand personal vision regarding the potential of well-being.

■ This exercise can be followed by a planning process that helps participants select specific ideas and focus on the formation of personal goals for positive behavior change.

TRAINER'S NOTES

WHOLE PERSON POTPOURRI
Creative Challenge List

 Select assignments from this list, alter as appropriate, or make up your own that fit the moment and the specific issues of the group you're working with. Be sure to have the materials needed for each challenge on hand and available for distribution with the assignment. Also collect a variety of odds and ends materials such as paper plates, cups, string, rubber bands, old clothes, magazines, cardboard boxes, sign standards, umbrellas, kazoos— anything that might enhance creativity. Put these resources in a central location for use by all groups as needed.

WHOLE PERSON TRIVIA

Using the Trivial Pursuit gameboard and pieces, design a game that demonstrates the whole person model of well-being.

Materials: *Trivial Pursuit game.*

WHOLE PERSON NURSING HOME

You are consultants to a national chain of nursing homes. Based on the variety of creative forces that energize people and help them regain and maintain wholeness, make recommendations for the policies and practices to be implemented for residents.

Materials: *Newsprint, markers, blank paper.*

HYMN FEST

Write a "Hymn to Wholeness." Use a common hymn tune and write as many whole person verses as you can in the time allowed. Be prepared to teach your hymn to the group and defend your recommendation that it become our national hymn. Write the final lyrics on newsprint so everyone can sing along.

Materials: *Newsprint, markers, blank paper.*

WHOLE PERSON WELLNESS GAME

Design a new game based on the concept of whole person wellness. The game should:

 1) actively involve everyone in this class;
 2) offer the experience of "diversity" in the whole as well as "unity " of the whole; and
 3) take 5 minutes or less to play

Materials: *Whatever is in the room.*

WHOLE PERSON GROUP EXERCISE

Design a total group exercise that demonstrates wholeness—body, mind, spirit, relationships. The exercise must involve every person in this session. Be prepared to lead the whole group through your design.

Materials: *None.*

WHOLE PERSON FIRST AID KIT

Design and present a whole person first aid kit—for use in physical, emotional, mental, spiritual and relational emergencies.

Materials: *Toy first aid kit.*

TOBACCO LOBBY

You are the Public Relations department for Philip Morris. Design and produce a 30-second TV commercial showing the American public that your company is already fully behind whole person wellness, and that your product helps move people toward wholeness. Use everyone in your group and be prepared to demonstrate.

Materials: *Whatever is in the room.*

TOT LOT

Using your Tinker Toy set, design and build a model piece of playground equipment that will help kids feel whole in all aspects of their being. Be prepared to demonstrate your invention and sell it to this workshop group.

Materials: *Set of Tinker Toys.*

CAPITOL HILL

You are the staff for your US senator. She is on a committee studying ways to improve our national health status. Prepare a background report suggesting recommendations she should make for changing federal policy and the positions she should take. Be sure to alert her to the resistance she will meet from various special interest groups as she tries to promote whole person well-being.

Materials: *Newsprint, markers, blank paper.*

BENEFITS PACKAGE

You are the bargaining team for the next AFL-CIO contract negotiations. Based on your vision of well-being and what helps people achieve wholeness, outline the full range of contract changes and fringe benefits you plan to seek.

Materials: *Newsprint, markers, blank paper.*

TONIGHT SHOW

You are writers for Johnny Carson. Prepare the opening monologue for his next show that focuses on the need for reaching wholeness and our cultural foibles and contradictions as we seek
· wholeness.

Materials: *Newsprint, markers, blank paper.*

VITALITY CALENDAR

Write a 30-day calendar of energizers—one-a-day suggestions guaranteed to double your vitality in one month. Be sure to include energizers from all five areas of life (check the newsprint sheets around the room for ideas). Be as creative and nutty as possible.

Materials: *Newsprint, markers, blank paper.*

FUTURE THINK TANK

Design the whole person clinic of the future. Based on the creative use of whole person energizers: Who will staff it? How will it operate? What happens for recipients of care? What prescriptions are offered? For your presentation to the whole group, draw up a floor plan and a description of services.

Materials: *Newsprint, markers, blank paper.*

WORKSHOP DESIGN

Design a one-day workshop in which participants will experience wholeness. Build in a full range of creative energizers in all dimensions so that participants have a truly whole person experience. Use the ideas generated earlier in the brainstorming as resources. Be prepared to announce your workshop to the entire group, complete with objectives, session outline and PR about why people should attend.

Materials: *Newsprint, markers, blank paper.*

GUIDED FANTASY

Write a 10-minute guided fantasy that helps people experience and move toward wholeness in their own life—body, mind, spirit, relationships, emotions.

Materials: *Newsprint, markers, blank paper.*

NIGHTLINE

You are the producers of ABC's "Nightline" with Ted Kopel. Design and orchestrate his next show featuring the concepts and controversies surrounding our search for wholeness. List your guests who will represent whole person well-being and your guests who will challenge it. Outline background notes and lead questions for Ted.

Materials: *Newsprint, markers, blank paper.*

MEDICAL JOURNAL

Write a sarcastic, tongue-in-cheek letter to the Editor of the *New England Journal of Medicine,*listing the high cost and grave dangers of the current popular cultural rush toward wholeness.

Materials: *Newsprint, markers, blank paper.*

52 PICK-ME-UP

Use this deck of cards to design a game or series of experiences that teaches whole person wellness—body, mind, spirit, relationships, vocation, emotions. Be sure that it involves everyone in the process and plan how you will demonstrate your game to the entire group.

Materials: *Deck of playing cards, newsprint, markers, blank paper, any other items in the room.*

WHOLISTIC HOTEL

The Hilton hotel chain has asked you to make recommendations for implementing the implications of the whole person model of well-being into the management of their hotel. Make recommendations on the total operation that will insure that guests check out more whole in every respect than when they checked in. Address issues such as: *1) facility alterations and use; 2) restaurant menus and atmosphere; 3) staff selection and training.*

Materials: *Newsprint, markers, blank paper.*

BIRTHDAY PARTY

Design a whole person birthday party for someone in this room. Be sure to celebrate physically, mentally, spiritually, interpersonally and emotionally with the birthday person!

Materials: *Birthday cake and candles, wrapping paper, ribbon, other items in the room.*

WELLNESS TOYS

You are the Research and Development think tank group for the Mattel toy company. Generate a list of new toys that would communicate the model of wholeness to kids. Describe each toy as fully as possible and develop a marketing strategy for each.

Materials: *Newsprint, markers, blank paper, other items in the room.*

WHOLE PERSON OF THE YEAR

Select a nationally known figure to receive the "Whole Person of the Year" award. Write the press release which outlines the qualities and achievements (body, mind, spirit, relationships) that distinguish this person for the award. You may opt for a "roast" approach if you wish, or play it straight.

Materials: *Newsprint, markers, blank paper.*

PRESCHOOL WELLNESS

Design the optimum preschool curriculum to be used by Headstart-type programs that will prepare young children as *whole persons* for their entrance into school. How will you approach physical, mental, emotional, spiritual, interpersonal and "wholistic" education?

Materials: *Newsprint, markers, blank paper.*

WHOLE PERSON LIBRARY

Redesign your public library (building and programs) into a laboratory of wholeness intended to promote vitality in all its dimensions.

Materials: *Newsprint, markers, blank paper*

117 HEALTH AND LIFESTYLE

The video **Health and Lifestyle** provides the centerpiece for a mini-workshop on various wellness topics.

GOALS

To provide an introduction to lifestyle issues related to health and wellness.

To identify personal habits that affect health and target specific lifestyle areas for change.

GROUP SIZE

Unlimited.

TIME FRAME

60–90 minutes

MATERIALS NEEDED

Health and Lifestyle Assessment worksheets for all; VCR and monitor; **Health and Lifestyle** video (28 minutes), available from The Altschul Group, 1560 Sherman Avenue, Suite 100, Evenston IL 60201. 800/421-2363 (Rental: $65.00 for VHS videocassette).

PROCESS

 This video provides an excellent overview of wellness concepts, including: what is wellness, risk factors for cardio-vascular disease, the role of lifestyle choices, reducing risk factors through healthy nutrition, stress management, exercise and habit control (smoking, eating, alchol use).

To design a session around the video, choose a particular emphasis (eg, cardiac risk factors, exercise, alcohol dependency, etc), then choose an appropriate icebreaker, planning process, group energizer and related assessment or skill builder exercise to supplement the video and highlight your area of concern. See the Variations for examples of other combinations using teaching designs from this and other volumes of the Stress and Wellness series. The process described here focuses on cardio-vascular risk factors and physical fitness using supplementary exercises from this volume.

1) The trainer begins with an icebreaker of her choice (eg, *Hearts at Risk, p 6*). (10–15 minutes)

2) After the group has warmed up to the topic and each other, the trainer shows the **Health and Lifestyle** video. (30 minutes)

☞ *About 14 minutes into the video, cardiologist Dr Herbert Benson describes his famous technique for managing stress—the Relaxation Response. For maximum learning and participant benefit, stop the film after this description (leave the lights off) and guide the group through 5 minutes or more of on the spot relaxation, repeating the steps outlined by Benson:*

+ *Sit quietly and comfortably in your chair with eyes closed.*
+ *Relax all the muscles of your body; start with your feet, head, neck, shoulders, hands, arms, and legs. Just let everything go loose.*
+ *Pay attention to your breathing; allow yourself to breathe slowly and naturally.*
+ *With each out-breath, say silently to yourself the word "one."*
+ *When other thoughts enter your mind, allow them to pass through and return your attention to your breathing and the word "me."*
+ *(After 5 or more minutes) sit quietly and slowly open your eyes . . . then slowly stretch.*

Allow a moment or two for re-acclimation before returning to the video.

3) When the video is over, the trainer asks participants to use a blank sheet of paper to record their responses to the video as she poses the following series of questions.

➤ First, I'd like you to think back over the video and recall the most memorable part for you. What caught your attention? Write down a brief description of whatever it is that made an impression on you.

➤ As you reflect on the video, what would you say was its message for you? Write down this key application for your life.

➤ Now turn to a neighbor and take a minute to tell each other about what it was in the video that struck you and something about why it made an impact on you. (2 minutes)

4) The trainer distributes **Health and Lifestyle Assessment** worksheets to everyone and leads the group step-by-step through the questions (which provide a review of the video content).

➤ In *Section A* mark *your risk factors for cardiovascular disease.* If you're not sure of any, then make a note to yourself about where you can find out the information.

➤ Research continues to support the concept that diet is a major contributor to lifestyle disease. In *Section B* make an *assessment of your diet* and then list changes you've already made and changes you still need to make if you want to move toward a healthier lifestyle.

➤ Stress was highlighted in the video as one of the key indirect risk factors for heart disease. In *Section C,* first assess your *overall stress level,* then mark how frequently you use the natural antidotes to the stress response—*exercise and relaxation.* Finally, take a look at the *seven qualities of people who manage stress well* and rank yourself on how consistently you use these strategies to manage your own stress.

➤ Consider for a moment *lifestyle habits* that affect your health and pick one that is potentially troublesome for you or one that you are having difficulty with (eg, alcohol, smoking, overeating, complaining, not expressing feelings, worrying, over-working, etc). Write this habit down in the top of *Section D.*

➤ How do you know this habit is a problem or potential problem? Does it displace more productive activities? Do you do it without thinking? Does it interfere with your judgment? Does it isolate you from others? Write down the symptoms that let you know this habit is problem-forming.

➤ Now consider how you developed this habit or dependency. Where did you learn the behavior? What supports or reinforces it? What are the cues? Consider whether this habit or dependency is something you want to change. What are some possible substitutes for this behavior that would give a healthier payoff? What would you have to stop or start doing to make such a change?

➤ If you don't want to change this habit right now, write a sentence or two describing why you are choosing to continue it.

➤ Finally, if you want to change this habit, jot some notes about how you might make the change (eg, quit in stages, stop cold turkey, get professional help, join a support group, etc).

5) The trainer instructs participants to form groups of 3 (or rejoin previous small groups) and spend 2–3 minutes each sharing reactions to the video and insights from their worksheets.

6) The trainer reconvenes the group and continues with the next content segment.

☞ *Take A Walk (p 52) provides a natural finale to this process since it offers immediate reinforcement for the health and lifestyle benefits of regular exercise.*

VARIATIONS

■ To design a special-focus presentation or workshop around this film, consult the suggestions below for icebreakers, planning processes, group energizers and other teaching designs from the Whole Person Handbooks series that might fit your theme and audience.

■ Whole Person Wellness Session:

Icebreakers: *Wellness Emblem (p 14); Two Minute Mill, Human Health/Illness Continuum (**Wellness 1**); Silent Auction (**Wellness 2**); Health-Oriented People Hunt (**Wellness 3**).*

Planning: *Real to Ideal (**Wellness 1**); Daily Wellness Graph (**Wellness 3**).*

Group Energizers: *12 Days of Wellness (p 113); Fit as a Fiddle (p 121); Noontime Energizers, Slogans and Bumper Stickers (**Wellness 1**); Cheers!, I'm Depressed! (**Wellness 2**); Limericks, Balancing Act (**Wellness 3**).*

Other: *Whole Person Health Appraisal, Wellness Congress (**Wellness 1**); Present Health Status, Wellness Wheel (**Wellness 3**); Well Cards, Health Lifelines (**Wellness 3**).*

■ Stress Management/Relaxation Focus

Icebreakers: *Attention to Tension (**Wellness 2**); Personal Stressors/ Copers (**Stress 1**); Life Event Bingo (**Stress 2**); Models (**Stress 3**); Wanted Posters (**Stress 4**).*

Planning: *One Step at a Time (**Stress 1**); Stress and Coping Journal (**Stress 2**); Change Pentagon (**Stress 3**); ABCDEFG Planner (**Stress 4**).*

Group Energizers: *60-Second Tension Tamers, Group Backrub (**Wellness 1**); Body Scanning, Good Morning World (**Wellness 2**); Get Off*

My Back (Stress 1); Seaweed and Oak (Stress 2); Merry-Go-Round, Human Knots (Stress 4).

Other: *AAAbc's of Stress Management, Stress Risk Factors, Unwinding (Stress 1); Circuit Overload (Stress 2); Recipe for Success, Lifetrap 3: Sick of Change (Stress 3); On the Job Stress Grid, Spider Web (Stress 4).*

■ Habit Control: Nutrition, Smoking, Alcohol Workshops

Icebreakers: *Lost and Found (p 4); Analogies (Wellness 1); Sabotage and Self-Care, Galloping Gourmet (Wellness 3).*

Planning: *Information Is Not Enough (p 93); Meet the New Me (Wellness 1); Cleaning Up My Act (Wellness 2).*

Group Energizers: *Twenty Reasons (p 132), On Purpose (p 127); Grabwell Grommet (Wellness 1); Ten Great Trips on Foot (Stress 1); 10-Second Break, The Garden (Stress 2); Kicking Your Stress Can-Can (Stress 3); Hot Tub (Stress 4).*

Other: *Letter from the Interior, Last Meal (Wellness 1); Medicine Cabinet, Lunch Duets (Wellness 2); Pileup Copers (Stress 2).*

■ Cardiovascular Disease Presentation

Icebreakers: *Wellness Goals/Health Concerns, Human Health/Illness Continuum (Wellness 1); Getting to Know You (Wellness 3).*

Planning: *Discoveries (p 100); Calorie Counter's Prayer (p 59); Shoulds, Wants, Wills (Wellness 1); One-A-Day Plan (Wellness 2); Chemical Independence, Consciousness-Raising Diet (Wellness 3); Goals, Obstacles, Actions (Stress 2); Imagine Success (Stress 3).*

Group Energizers: *As the Seasons Turn (p 116); Singalong 1 (Wellness 1); Singalong 2 (Stress 1); Treasure Chest (Stress 2); What's the Hurry?, Chinese Swing (Stress 3).*

Other: *Lifetrap 1: Workaholism (Stress 1); Four Corners, Marathon Strategy (Wellness 1); Investing in Health, Personal Fitness Check (Wellness 2); Fit to be Interviewed (Wellness 3).*

HEALTH AND LIFESTYLE ASSESSMENT

A. MY RISK FACTORS

___ high blood pressure ___ cholesterol levels   ___ smoking
___ dietary excesses   ___ lack of exercise   ___ overweight
      (fat, salt, sugar)   ___ chronic stress   ___ alcohol abuse

B. NUTRITION

1. My diet today is:

___ healthier   ___ about the same   ___ less healthy than 5 years ago.
___ healthier   ___ about the same   ___ less healthy than 1 year ago.
___ healthier   ___ about the same   ___ less healthy than 1 week ago.

2. Positive changes I've made: 3. Changes I need to make:

C. STRESS MANAGEMENT

1. My stress level is: ___ low   ___ medium   ___ high

2. To counteract the stress response: N = Never; S = Sometimes;
                                            O = Often; A = Almost Always

I substitute exercise to discharge the tension   N   S   O   A
I use relaxation techniques to let go.   N   S   O   A

3. Characteristics I share with people who manage stress well:

I enjoy moments of solitude every day.   N   S   O   A
I use humor and play to change my mood.   N   S   O   A
I have close ties with family and friends.   N   S   O   A
I engage in absorbing pastimes.   N   S   O   A
I am able to tolerate frustration.   N   S   O   A
I handle criticism without falling apart.   N   S   O   A
I unschedule my life when it gets too hectic.   N   S   O   A

D. MY NEGATIVE
LIFESTYLE HABIT _____

How is it a problem for you?

How did it develop?

Possible substitutes:

How would you like to change?

118 WELLNESS PHILOSOPHY

In this exercise, each participant creates a personal credo of wellness and presents that philosophical statement to the group.

GOALS

To examine the concept of wellness as set forth by pioneers in the field.

To create a personal definition of wellness.

GROUP SIZE

Unlimited.

TIME FRAME

20–30 minutes

MATERIALS NEEDED

Wellness Is and **My Wellness Message** worksheets for each participant.

PROCESS

1) The trainer introduces the exercise by outlining the wellness philosophy articulated by "experts" in the field.

   - John W Travis, a physician from Mill Valley, California, is one of the pioneers in the wellness field. Dr Travis believes that **wellness is everyone's right, privilege and responsibility.**

   - **Wellness is a process, not a state.** We don't "achieve" it, but rather move back and forth on a continuum ranging from "low level worseness" to "high level wellness"—a term invented by another wellness pioneer, Donald B Ardell.

   - Ardell believes that **high level wellness is characterized by** positive self-esteem, a sense of purpose, acceptance of self and others, appreciation of peak experiences, integrity and competence, creativity, sense of humor, easy expression of affection and feelings, commitment to excellence, clear value orientation, infrequent illness, high level of fitness, and freedom from negative addictions.

   - Travis believes that **the key cornerstones of wellness are self-responsibility and love.** Self-responsibility begins with your awareness of self—body, mind, spirit, relationships—and ends with deliberate choice-making and action for well-being. Love means trusting that you have the resources to respond to life's challenges (including illness) as opportunities to grow, accepting yourself and celebrating the worth of all persons.

● Ardell, Travis and other wellness experts also believe that wellness is a personal issue. **Each of us is the ultimate "expert" on our own well-being.** We take the best of others' ideas and integrate it with our own principles and experiences to formulate a personal philosophy of wellness that guides our self-care choices.

2) The trainer distributes **Wellness Is** worksheets and guides participants through the process of developing a personal statement about wellness.

➤ Add your name to the by-line beside John Travis. When you're finished, you'll be the co-author of your personal wellness definition.

➤ If you agree with a statement, leave it the way it is. If you wholeheartedly agree, you may want to emphasize it with underlining, stars or some other symbol.

➤ If you *disagree strongly* with a statement, cross it out.

➤ If you think a statement *should be revised,* cross out or add words until it reads the way you want it to read.

➤ If you think an important element of the definition has been *left out,* add it at the bottom of the sheet.

3) After about 5 minutes the trainer distributes **My Wellness Message** worksheets and gives directions for creating a personal wellness message.

➤ Now it's your turn to become the innovators who will create a new definition of wellness. Write your name at the top of the worksheet, next to the word "By."

➤ You will have three minutes to prepare a *one-minute presentation* on wellness for the rest of your group. You can use one or more of the idea starters at the top of the worksheet for your theme, or you can create your own angle.

➤ Be creative and sincere. The most successful speakers are the ones who can say something original, interesting and believable.

☞ *If participants are reluctant to speak in front of the group, remind them that it's only for one minute. Encourage bolder members of the group to go first. Exhort everyone to be supportive of others as they make their presentations.*

4) The trainer allows three minutes for participants to prepare their presentations. Then each participant is given a minute to make a presentation.

5) After the presentations, the trainer asks group members to choose the "award winners" for "Most Innovative" and "Most Likely to Succeed as a Wellness Expert."

> ☞ *Keep this portion light—no secret ballots or popularity contests. The point is to encourage participants to discuss each other's presentations for a couple of minutes.*

6) The trainer closes with a reminder about self-responsibility.

- Instead of looking to outside events for answers or motivation in our search for health and wholeness, we need to look inside ourselves to determine what we need—and then take action on our own behalf. We then can consult the "experts" without giving them the responsibility for our well-being.

VARIATION

- With more than 15 participants, divide into small groups (6–10 people) for the presentations in *Step 4*. As part of *Step 5*, award winners from each small group could make their presentation to the entire group.

Chalktalk notes and wellness definitions adapted from John Travis' excellent **Wellness Workbook** *(Berkeley CA: Ten Speed Press, 1981, 1988) and Don Ardell's classic,* **High Level Wellness** *(Berkeley CA: Ten Speed Press, 1977, 1986).*

WELLNESS IS . . .

By: John W Travis, MD, and _____

■ Knowing what your real needs are and how to get them met;

■ Expressing emotions in ways that communicate to other people what you are experiencing;

■ Acting assertively, and not passively or aggressively;

■ Enjoying your body by means of adequate nutrition, exercise and physical awareness;

■ Being engaged in projects that are meaningful to you and reflect your most important inner values;

■ Knowing how to create and cultivate close relationships with others;

■ Responding to challenges in life as opportunities to grow in strength and maturity, rather than feeling beset by "problems";

■ Creating the life you really want, rather than just reacting to what "seems to happen";

■ Relating to troublesome physical symptoms in ways that bring improvement in your condition as well as increased knowledge about yourself;

■ Enjoying a basic sense of well-being, even through times of adversity;

■ Knowing your own inner patterns—emotional and physical—and understanding "signals" your body gives you;

■ Trusting that your own personal resources are your greatest strength for living and growing;

■ Knowing you are not separate from other people, the earth, divinity;

■ Experiencing yourself as a wonderful person.

MY WELLNESS MESSAGE TO THE WORLD
By: _____

IDEA STARTERS

The components of wellness are . . .
The real core of wellness is . . .
People need to change their thinking by . . .
The turning point for me was . . .
The aspect of wellness most often overlooked is . . .
If I were a "wellness expert," I would tell people . . .

YOUR MESSAGE:

119 SYMPHONY OF THE CELLS

In this two-part exercise, participants get a "cellular" view of the various physical and non-physical body systems and explore how each system contributes to the overall harmony of the whole person.

GOALS

To provide an imaginative and fun introduction to the "whole person" concept of well-being.

To introduce the concept of physical and non-physical body systems working together for total well-being.

GROUP SIZE

This exercise works best with a group of 40 or more, but can be adapted for smaller groups.

TIME FRAME

20–30 minutes, longer with larger groups.

MATERIALS NEEDED

Newsprint sheets posted at locations around the room corresponding to each physical and non-physical system (3 sheets and a marker at each location); Large sign for each physical system (respiratory, cardiac, digestive, genital/urinary, musculo-skeletal, neurological/sensory);Large sign with symbol for each non-physical system (heart, light bulb, hand or arrow, candle); Nametags with "cell" names and symbols.

☞ *In this exercise nametags are used twice to organize participants into small groups with different people. Make up nametags in advance. Each nametag should have the **name of a body system** (respiratory, cardiac, digestive, genital/urinary, musculo-skeletal, neurological/sensory) and a **symbol** for a whole person **non-physical system** (emotional [heart], mental [light bulb], social [hand or arrows], spiritual [candle]).*

Make sure that people are in a group with different people during the second round. Nametags with the same body system (eg, digestive) should have a variety of non-physical system symbols (eg, hand, heart, candle, etc).

PROCESS

A. Exploring Body Systems (10–15 minutes)

1) When participants enter the room, the trainer instructs them to pick up a nametag (prepared with the system names and symbols), write their name on it, and wear it throughout the exercise.

2) The trainer introduces the exercise by describing the function of cells in the human body, emphasizing the following points:

   ● Different types of cells make up our physical systems, which all work together for overall physical well-being.

   ● Each physical system has a role to play, and no one system can survive on its own. We can think of a well-functioning body as a symphony, where each instrument follows its own score, but all work together for a harmonious whole.

   ● No matter how healthy a single system is, it relies on the health and good functioning of all other systems for total physical well-being.

     ☞ *If the rest of the session will focus on a single system (eg, cardiovascular), you may wish to emphasize that system during this introduction.*

3) The trainer tells participants that each of them is a "cell" belonging to a physical system, as noted on their nametags. He instructs participants to gather with their fellow-cells near the signs indicating their *physical systems.*

   ☞ *If time permits, or if this process is used as a get-acquainted exercise, you may omit posting the signs and allow people to mill around looking for the other "cells" in their systems. When the systems are assembled, give them sheets of newsprint and a marker.*

4) The trainer instructs each group of "cells" to consider their *function.*

   ➤ Brainstorm together about what your physical system contributes to the overall well-being of the body.

   ➤ Someone should volunteer to be the recorder for your group and keep track of all ideas on one of the newsprint sheets.

     ☞ *Allow about 2 minutes for this discussion, then announce the next step.*

   ➤ Decide together on your major contribution to the body and circle it on the newsprint.

5) As soon as groups have reached a decision, the trainer asks the "cell systems" to shift their focus slightly for another round of self- exploration.

➤ Take another 2 minutes to discuss together what the cells in your body system *need* from the rest of the body systems in order to stay healthy and to function well.

➤ Record your ideas on the second newsprint.

☞ *Pause 2–3 minutes, then pose the summary question.*

➤ Decide together on your most overriding need and circle it.

6) The trainer challenges each "system" to figure out a way to represent itself as a body system through sound and motion.

☞ *Announce that groups will have 3 minutes to decide on and practice their sound and motion. If necessary, suggest that each person could make the same motion, or cells could create a moving group sculpture of their organ system.*

7) The trainer asks all groups to practice their sounds and motions simultaneously. This is the dress rehearsal for the "symphony of the cells"—the sound of a healthy body.

8) The trainer calls on each group to make an individual presentation of their system.

➤ First, perform your sound and motion. If necessary, explain to us what it means.

➤ Second, tell us about your most important contribution to the overall well-being of the body.

➤ Finally, what do you most need from the rest of the body?

☞ *After all systems have made their presentations, you may want to have a final unison performance of the "symphony of the cells."*

B. Whole Person Well-Being (15 minutes)

9) The trainer introduces the second part of the exercise by emphasizing the following points:

● Most ancient civilizations realized that there is no real dividing line between physical and non-physical systems. What affects one, affects the other.

©1994 Whole Person Press 210 W Michigan Duluth MN 55802   (800) 247-6789

● The wellness movement is built around the concept that we must function as whole beings if we are to function at our best. We've just looked at the systems that make up our physical self; now we'll do the same for the non-physical systems.

10) The trainer tells participants to form new groups, gathering with fellow "cells" in their non-physical systems under the signs that match the symbols on their nametags.

☞ *You may want to point out the locations and explain the symbols and systems again.*

11) The trainer challenges each "system" of "cells" to write a definition of their system that describes the **components** and **functions** of that system.

☞ *Give a few examples (eg, mental components could include curiosity, intelligence, logic, attitudes, etc; spiritual functions could be to provide hope, to cope with loss, to choose values, to give meaning, etc), but don't overdo it! Let the groups struggle with the issue and tap into their own creativity.*

12) After 2–3 minutes the trainer interrupts and instructs groups to write their definition on newsprint.

13) *Steps 4 and 5 are repeated, with groups brainstorming **what their system contributes** to the overall well-being of the person and deciding **what their system needs most** from the other physical and non-physical systems. (5–8 minutes in all)*

14) The trainer announces that each "system" has 3 minutes to decide on a sound and motion combination that represents itself.

15) The trainer asks all groups to perform their sounds and motions simultaneously. (Another "symphony of the cells!")

16) The trainer invites each group to introduce their system to the rest of the whole person.

➤ First, perform your sound and motion. If necessary, explain to us what it means.

➤ Second, tell us the definition of your system.

➤ Third, tell us how your system contributes to whole person wellness.

➤ Finally, what do you most need from the person in order to function well?

©1994 Whole Person Press 210 W Michigan Duluth MN 55802   (800) 247-6789

17) The trainer uses the information generated by the group activities to make a closing summary about the importance of both physical and non-physical systems for whole person well-being.

VARIATIONS

■ If time is limited, do just one half of the exercise (ie, either the physical or the non-physical systems). The trainer makes the point that systems work together for total well-being.

■ Instead of using different physical systems, divide the group into different parts of one system. If the day's sessions focus on heart disease, for example, "cells" could be assigned to different parts of the circulatory system—the heart muscle, the blood vessels within the heart, the other blood vessels in the body, etc.

■ A smaller group (15 or fewer) can examine each system in turn, rather than dividing up into separate groups.

TRAINER'S NOTES

Self-Care
Strategies

120 DECADES

Participants review their experiences with illness and self-care habits in different periods of their life.

GOALS

To review personal health history.

To uncover self-care patterns.

GROUP SIZE

Unlimited.

TIME FRAME

15–20 minutes

MATERIALS NEEDED

Health History worksheets for all.

PROCESS

1) The trainer distributes **Health History** worksheets to all participants and invites them to focus on the first box: *Preschool Years.*

   ➤ Think back on the years before you started school. Where did you live? What was happening in your family? In your neighborhood?

   ➤ Narrow your focus now and recall what health issues were important during those early years of life. Were there any problems associated with your birth? Were you a colicky baby? Did you have an ear infection or other chronic illnesses? Were you the picture of health? How about accidents? Jot down any health issues that you know of from that period of your life.

   ➤ Next, try to remember what responsibilities you took for your own well-being. Did you eat well? Sleep enough? Exercise regularly? Wear your boots? etc. Jot down any self-care actions for health.

2) The trainer guides the group through each of the *decade* boxes on the worksheet, adapting the sequence of questions from *Step 1* with appropriate examples to fit each decade.

©1994 Whole Person Press 210 W Michigan Duluth MN 55802   (800) 247-6789

☞ *Keep the pace brisk, or this process will bog down. But make sure people have time to get beneath their flip surface responses.*

When you get to decades participants have not yet reached, invite people to answer the question with what they imagine will be true for them, based on what they have noticed about family and friends in those age groups.

➤ Where were you during this time period?

➤ What health issues affected your life during this decade?

☞ *Highlight typical issues for the age group such as:*

grade school: *accidents, shots, allergies, chicken pox, body size, glasses, coordination.*

junior/senior high: *acne, weight control, body image, growing pains, menstruation, sexuality, alcohol, athletic injuries, headaches, digestive upsets, braces.*

young adult: *contraception, mono, alcohol and drugs, pregnancy, childbirth, sexually transmitted diseases.*

25–35: *stress, physical fitness, birth control, conception, smoking, spare tire.*

35–45: *blood pressure, eyesight, mid-life crisis.*

45–55: *heart disease, hormone replacement, cancer, cosmetic surgery.*

55–65: *hearing loss, heart attacks, cholesterol level, dentures, depression.*

65+: *sleep disturbances, grief, medication, loss of memory, boredom, physical limitations.*

➤ What positve self-care habits did you develop or continue during that period? How did you take care of yourself?

3) The trainer divides participants into groups according to the year they graduated from high school.

☞ *Adapt the range of years so that there are 4–7 people in each group.*

4) After groups are settled, the trainer instructs participants to spend 2–3 mintues describing to the group what they learned about their health and self-care patterns over the decades.

HEALTH HISTORY

PRESCHOOL	GRADE SCHOOL	JR/SR HIGH
health issues self-care	health issues self-care	health issues self-care
18–25	**25–35**	**35-45**
health issues self-care	health issues self-care	health issues self-care
45–55	**55–65**	**65 +**
health issues self-care	health issues self-care	health issues self-care

©1994 Whole Person Press 210 W Michigan Duluth MN 55802   (800) 247-6789

121 TAKE A WALK!

This exercise gives new meaning to the term "active learning"—as participants take a twenty-minute walk and compare notes on their experiences.

GOALS

To exercise for twenty minutes.

To explore potential supports for beginning and continuing a walking program.

To demonstrate that creativity can spice up an everyday activity and make it more appealing.

GROUP SIZE

Unlimited.

TIME FRAME

45–60 minutes

MATERIALS NEEDED

Blackboard or newsprint easel; **Eight-Week Take-a-Walk Program** handouts for all; one of the **Take-a-Walk Assignments** for each pair: headphone radio, basketball, aluminum can.

☞ *Before the session photocopy the Assignment list on pp 56–57 and cut it up so that you have one assignment for each pair. Or write them on index cards. Feel free to invent other assignments that relate to the overall theme of your session or that particularly fit your environment (eg, pick up trash in the city, leaves in the wilderness). The point is to add a creative dimension to the walking experience.*

PROCESS

1) The trainer introduces the concept of walking as an easy, natural activity that can also be an excellent aerobic exercise and calorie-burner.

2) The trainer polls the group on their walking attitudes and patterns by asking for a show of hands on the following questions:

✔ Do you think a regular walking program would benefit your health?

✔ Have you ever walked for exercise or enjoyment?

✔ Have you taken a walk of 15 minutes or longer in the past week?

3) The trainer asks the group to give examples of what has in the past stopped them from from taking a walk (eg, the weather, don't have the right shoes/clothes, it's boring, don't have the time). He records on the board all the barriers and excuses mentioned.

☞ *If no one mentions time, add it to the list yourself before the next step.*

4) The trainer acknowledges that it may be hard to find time in a busy schedule for walking. He announces that time will not be a problem today, because the group is going to go for a walk right now!

5) The trainer gives general directions for the walk.

➤ First, pair up with someone you would like as a walking companion.

☞ *Make sure everyone has a partner (and only one!) before describing the next step. If there is an extra person, pair up with him and take a walk yourself!*

➤ You will be taking a walk together, following these guidelines:
   ➤ Take a minute or two to warm up as you leave the building by walking slowly for about a block.
   ➤ Then walk briskly for 10 minutes.
   ➤ Turn around and walk briskly back. (10 minutes)
   ➤ Take 1–2 minutes to cool down (walk slowly) before coming back in the building.

☞ *If people are wearing inappropriate shoes for walking, tell them that they're only going to walk for twenty minutes, and they can go more slowly if their shoes demand it. Everyone should be able to keep moving, no matter how slowly, for twenty minutes.*

6) The trainer instructs participants to take their resting pulse rate (count 10 seconds and multiply by 6) and write it down.

☞ *Try to make sure that each pair has a watch with a second hand so they can take their pulse rate again at the turnaround point, and when they return.*

7) The trainer announces the special nature of this *Take A Walk* routine and distributes an assignment to each pair.

☞ *If you think of other assignments, perhaps ones that tie into the theme of the session, use those instead. Just make sure that there are enough different assignments so teams can compare notes on their different experiences when they return.*

➤ Decide who will be *Reebok* and who will be *Adidas*.

➤ This is going to be a creative "walkabout" designed to overcome some of the obstacles to walking we talked about earlier (eg, boredom, isolation, etc). Each pair has an unusual task to accomplish during your walk.

8) The trainer sends the pairs out for their walk. All pairs should start their walks at the same time.

☞ *If it is cold or wet outside, give the group members a few minutes to get their coats, boots and other wraps. Make the point that walking is an all-weather activity. Then send them on their way.*

9) As the pairs return, the trainer reminds people to record their pulse rates and then immediately assigns pairs to discussion groups of six people (3 pairs). Groups spend 5–10 minutes comparing notes on their assignments and talking about what they learned on their walks.

10) When all groups have returned and had at least a few minutes to share their experiences, the trainer instructs them to spend 2–3 minutes brainstorming a list of ideas for increasing the likelihood that they could be successful in starting and maintaining their own walking program. The list should be based on their experiences during today's walk.

At the end of the time, the trainer asks each group to decide on their *five favorite supports* from the list they generated.

11) The trainer brings the entire group back together for reports from the small groups. Each group describes briefly the walking assignments of the people in that group, then shares their list of factors for success. The trainer writes down the most important supports as they are mentioned and uses these examples to illustrate a summary of principles for enhancing a personal walking program.

● Try both competition and cooperation.

● Use your imagination. Meditate. Fantasize.

● Involve all your senses.

● Make it fun! Adopt a childlike attitude.

● Listen to your body's signals. Learn to tolerate physical discomfort.

● Use affirmations to picture yourself as a vital, physically fit person.

12) The trainer distributes **Eight-Week Take-A-Walk Program** handouts and reviews the program with participants as part of a closing chalktalk on the benefits of walking.

- **Walking is safe exercise, with almost no risk of injury.** Virtually all physicians would endorse a walking program—no matter what your fitness level.

- **A regular walking program can help you control your weight while you increase your cardiovascular fitness.** It's also an ideal exercise for women who want to prevent osteoporosis and for couples and families who want to spend healthy time together.

- **You need to walk 3–4 times a week to become fit and stay fit.** Taking every other day off gives your body a chance to rest and recover and reduces the chances of injury. Walking that's done on the job doesn't count. It's not vigorous enough or sustained enough for cardiovascular fitness.

- **Walking is natural**—it doesn't require new skills. It's a sport you can practice alone or with friends, anywhere, for a life-time. **So, take a walk!**

VARIATION

■ In a day-long workshop, combine this exercise with the lunch break as a healthy model for integrating exercise into the workday.

TAKE-A-WALK ASSIGNMENTS

Reebok listens to a headphone radio while *Adidas* acts as a "guardian angel" to protect your partner from traffic, pedestrians, etc. Switch roles at the turnaround point.

> *Take your pulse at the turnaround point*

During your walk, you will take turns tuning in to messages from your body and verbalizing each awareness to your partner. During the first half, *Reebok* keeps up a steady stream of chatter, describing in detail every body sensation. *Adidas* should listen and encourage non-verbally. Change roles at the turnaround point.

> *Take your pulse at the turnaround point*

During the first half of your walk, compare notes on your experiences in junior high school (eg, building, teachers, sports, dating, favorite subjects, fads, music, etc). At the halfway point, separate and walk back along different routes or on opposite sides of the street.

> *Take your pulse at the turnaround point*

Your job is to count how many steps you take during this walk. If your strides are similar, walk in unison and count out loud together. If not, each person should mentally count her or his own steps. The counting is a form of meditation; focus on the numbers and the rhythm.

> *Take your pulse at the turnaround point*

Your job during this walk is to tell each other all the nursery rhymes, jump-rope chants, cheers and other word/rhythms you can remember. See if you can make the words match the rhythm of your strides. When you run out of ideas, start over again or pick one or two favorites to repeat so that your whole walk is accompanied by these childhood chants.

> *Take your pulse at the turnaround point*

The object of this walk is to clear your mind as you exercise your body. During the first half of the walk, *Reebok* should pay attention to whatever thoughts enter your mind. As you become aware of each thought, verbalize it to your partner and then tune in to your mental processes again. You will probably have a steady stream of unrelated thoughts ("I'm tired . . . I wonder what will happen when we get back . . . I forgot to pick up the laundry . . . What time is it?"). Just say out loud everything that comes to your mind. Switch roles at the midpoint of your walk.

> *Take your pulse at the turnaround point*

During your walk, play one or more games together. Possibilities: the *Alphabet Game* (find letters of the alphabet in order on signs), *I Spy* (one person picks out a visible object and tells its color, partner guesses what it is), *20 Questions.*

> *Take your pulse at the turnaround point*

This walk will be an adventure in giving up control. Take along a coin. On the way out, flip the coin twice at **each corner** to determine your direction. *Flip 1: heads = straight, tails = turn. Flip 2 (for direction): heads = left, tails = right.* If the neighborhood is unfamiliar, be sure you have pen and paper to make a map so you can find your way back along the same route.

> *Take your pulse at the turnaround point*

Take an aluminum can on your walk. Your assignment is to play *Kick the Can* together for the full 20 minutes. Take turns kicking — and watch out for traffic!

> *Take your pulse at the turnaround point*

You will need a basketball for your walk. Imagine that the two of you are in the *NBA Annual Pairs Walk & Dribble Contest.* There are three rules: a) the ball must be bouncing at all times (except when crossing the street);   b) you must alternate responsibility for dribbling;   c) each person should dribble at least 3 bounces and not more than 10 bounces before bounce-passing the ball to your partner. Be careful!

> *Take your pulse at the turnaround point*

Adidas and **Reebok** are neck-and-neck for the gold medal in the *50-kilometer race-walking event in the Olympics.* It's not just speed that counts in this event; it's form, concentration, and evenness of pace. As you walk, imagine the crowds cheering. Don't go too fast, but keep up a good, steady pace. Like any top athlete, concentrate on what you're doing and also on what your competitor is doing. If you like, talk and compare notes as you race for the gold medal.

> *Take your pulse at the turnaround point*

Imagine that the two of you are the honor guard leading a parade for a hero's homecoming. You are wearing impressive dress uniforms. If you like, you can hum, whistle or sing marching songs.

> *Take your pulse at the turnaround point*

EIGHT-WEEK TAKE-A-WALK PROGRAM

☞ *Before you start: Shoes are a walker's best friend. There should be 1/2"
to 3/4" of space between your longest toe and the end of the shoe. Soles
should be flexible and somewhat bouncy. This walking program is based
on the book, Walking: The Pleasure Exercise, by Mort Malkin (Rodale
Press, 1986).*

Week 1: Walk for 10 minutes (continuously!) every other day.
*If you miss a day, walk the next day instead. Set aside a special
time just for walking. Don't try to combine it with other activities.*

Week 2: Walk for 15 minutes (continuously) every other day.
*Start Week 2 immediately after Week 1. This means you'll walk
three days one week, four days the next. Walk as briskly as you
can. Walk as if you're proud of what you're doing—you should be!*

Week 3: Walk for 22 minutes every other day. Keep a brisk pace.
*Warm up by walking at a slow pace for a few minutes. This does
not count as part of the 22-minute workout.*

Week 4: Walk for 33 minutes every other day. Continue a brisk pace.
*Pay attention to form. The heel strikes the ground first, then the
foot rolls forward and pushes off on the toe. Feet should follow
each other in a straight line.*

Week 5: Walk for 45 minutes every other day.
*In addition to warming up, cool down after your walk by walking
slowly for a few minutes, then stretching slowly, holding each
stretch for 30 seconds, and releasing slowly.*

Week 6: Walk briskly for 45 minutes every other day.
*Try to increase your pace, but keep the pace even. If you can't
keep up the pace you set at the beginning of your walk, slow
down, but don't stop. Keep moving for the entire 45 minutes.*

Week 7: Walk briskly for 1 hour every other day.
*To keep up the challenge, measure the distance you cover. Walk
a measured course, or walk on a track.*

Week 8: Walk very briskly for 1 hour every other day. Repeat this
schedule for upcoming weeks.
*"Very brisk" means that you should feel as if you are pushing
yourself a bit. You should be breathing hard but still able to carry
on a conversation.*

122 CALORIE COUNTER'S PRAYER

This exercise combines humor and meaning by using the 23rd Psalm as a metaphor for weight loss. Participants write their own "Personal Psalm" for behavior change.

GOALS

To encourage group members to write a Personal Psalm for wellness.

To use a familiar and meaningful format for a humorous approach to behavior change.

GROUP SIZE

Unlimited.

TIME FRAME

10–15 minutes

MATERIALS NEEDED

The Calorie Counter's Prayer script; **Personal Psalm** worksheets for all.

PROCESS

1) The trainer introduces the **Calorie Counter's Prayer** and reads it aloud to the group.

   ☞ *In introducing the prayer, you may wish to say that it is not intended to offend anyone. Sometimes things that are very familiar and meaningful can help us see difficult issues in a different light. At the same time, humor can help us get a new perspective on a topic like being overweight, which often makes us feel guilty or inadequate. If we can see the lighter side, we'll have a better chance of changing our behavior patterns.*

2) The trainer distributes a **Personal Psalm** worksheet to each participant and invites people to fill it out for themselves. (5 minutes)

3) The trainer uses the prayers as a bridge to a more in-depth presentation on nutrition or eating habits (eg, *Last Meal, **Wellness 1**; Lunch Duets, **Wellness 2**; Consciousness Raising Diet, **Wellness 3**).

VARIATIONS

■ Focus the content of the Personal Psalm on a different area of well-being such as exercise, stress, whole-person wellness, etc.

■ The trainer may divide participants into groups of three and ask them to discuss their Personal Psalms with each other.

■ If the group is particularly close-knit or open, the trainer may ask for people to read their Personal Psalms aloud.

THE CALORIE COUNTER'S PRAYER Script

The Lord is my shepherd, I shall not want.
He maketh me to lie down and do push-ups.
He giveth me sodium-free bread,
He restoreth my waistline.
He leadeth me past the refrigerator, for my own sake.
He maketh me to partake of green beans instead of potatoes.
He leadeth me past the pizzeria.

Yea, though I walk through the bakery,
I shall not falter, for Thou art with me;
Thy diet colas, they comfort me.
Thou preparest a diet for me in the presence of mine enemies,
Thou annointest my lettuce with low-cal oil.
My cup will not overflow.

Surely Ry-Krisp and D-Zerta shall follow me all the days of my life,
And I will live with pangs of hunger forever.

*This prayer is a perenniel favorite in **Dear Abby**.*

My Personal Psalm for Wellness

The Lord is my shepherd, I shall not want.

He maketh me _____ ,

He giveth me _____ ,

He restoreth _____ .

He leadeth me _____

for mine own sake.

He maketh me _____ .

He leadeth me _____ .

Yea, though I walk _____ ,

I shall _____ ,

for Thou art with me;

Thy _____ and Thy _____

they comfort me.

Thou preparest a _____ for me

in the presence of _____ ,

Thou anointest my _____ with _____ .

My cup _____ .

Surely _____ and _____

shall follow me all the days of my life and I will

_____ forever.

©1994 Whole Person Press 210 W Michigan Duluth MN 55802   (800) 247-6789

123 SELF-ESTEEM GRID

In this assessment of a key component of health, participants affirm their extra-ordinary qualities, rank themselves on characteristics of high and low self-esteem and make plans to boost their self-image.

GOALS

To explore the role of self-esteem in whole person well-being.

To assess self-esteem and affirm personal strengths.

To identify priorities for self-improvement.

GROUP SIZE

Unlimited.

TIME FRAME

45–50 minutes

MATERIALS NEEDED

Characteristics of Low Self-Esteem and **Characteristics of High Self-Esteem** worksheets for all.

PROCESS

1) The trainer asks participants to pair up with a neighbor for an experiment in self-esteem.

   ➤ All of us in this room are quite extraordinary people! Even though we often feel very ordinary, each of us is unique in a whole host of ways. Your task during the next few minutes is to think of all the different ways that you are not ordinary.

   ➤ Think about your physical appearance, your attitudes, your job training, your skills, your interests, difficult or challenging life experiences you have weathered, contributions you make in your job or community, special knowledge, etc. In what ways are you extra-ordinary (better/worse/different from other people)?

   ➤ You will have 2 minutes each to convince your partner that you are not an ordinary person by listing all the ways that you are extra-ordinary! The person with the smaller hat size should begin. I will tell you when to switch.

☞ *Interrupt after 2 minutes and instruct the second partner to list his extraordinary qualities. After the second person has talked for 2 minutes, call time and ask if anyone got a swelled head from so much bragging.*

2) The trainer asks for reactions and observations from the group. She uses these insights as a springboard for a brief chalktalk on the importance of positive self-esteem in a wellness lifestyle.

- **Self-esteem is the key to wellness.** If you don't believe you are a valuable, worthwhile person, you won't believe that wellness is your right and privilege—and you're not likely to take good care of yourself.

- If you don't respect yourself and believe in your capabilities, you won't take responsibility for your own well-being and make the necessary choices and changes for health. If you don't trust your own resources, you're likely to depend too much on others for answers instead of looking inside yourself and trusting that you know what's best for you.

- If you feel powerless and inadequate, you can hardly be assertive about your rights and needs. If you don't think you're an interesting person, you won't seek out relationships and reach out to others who could support and affirm you.

- **These common sense notions are supported by research.** In a 1979 study by the California Department of Health, researchers documented that high self-esteem and a sense of control over one's destiny are positively related to mental and physical well-being. People with a healthy self-esteem believe that they have the resources to cope with whatever life may hold for them—and they do!

3) The trainer distributes **Characteristics of Low Self-Esteem** worksheets to participants and guides them through the assessment.

☞ *Don't rush this process. Give plenty of examples along the way and pause between steps so participants can thoughtfully consider their assessment.*

➤ This list includes 25 characteristics that are often associated with low self-esteem. Read through the list and consider each quality. Does this description fit you? To what degree? Do you ever feel this way? How often? As you make your assessment, use a 1 to 10 scale:

1 = not at all characteristic of me;
10 = extremely characteristic of me.

➤ In *Column A* mark where you would rank yourself *today* on each characteristic, using the 1 to 10 scale.

➤ In *Column B* mark where you would have ranked yourself *five years ago,* using the same scale.

➤ Look over your list and reflect on the changes that have occurred over time and potential changes you would like to make for the future.

    ➤ Have you improved over the last five years in any areas? In *Column C* put a check by those areas which are *less true* for you now than they were five years ago.

    ➤ Put an X in *Column C* by the four *areas you would most like to improve* in the next year.

    ➤ Then *circle* the quality you consider most important to change.

➤ At the bottom of the worksheet in *Section D* list at least *three steps you could take to change that perception* of yourself and the related feelings and behaviors.

➤ Finally, complete the sentence in *Section E.*

4) The trainer distributes copies of the **Characteristics of High Self-Esteem** worksheet and announces that the second "quiz" may be much more difficult since most people find it easier to acknowledge their inadequacies than to affirm their adequacies.

She invites participants to assess their self-esteem from another perspective and guides them through the worksheet.

    ☞ *Don't rush. For maximum benefit this sequence of questions should take 10-15 minutes for participants to answer.*

➤ This list includes qualities and behaviors that are commonly associated with positive self-esteem. Read through the list and consider how true each item is for you. Again, use the 1 to 10 scale as you assess the degree to which this description fits you:

    1 = not at all characteristic of me;
    10 = extremely characteristic of me.

➤ In *Column F,* mark where you would rank yourself on each quality *today,* using the 1 to 10 scale.

➤ In *Column G,* mark where you would have ranked yourself *five years ago.*

➤ Look over the list again. Have you made some improvements over the years?

    ➤ In Column H, *check* those areas where your self-esteem has blossomed.

➤ Mark with an X the *four areas you would most like to improve* or focus on

➤ Then *circle* the most important one.

▶ Now, at the bottom of the worksheet in *Section J*, list at least three ways you could develop that quality and enhance your self-esteem.

▶ Finally, complete the sentence in *Section K*.

5) The trainer invites participants to pair up with their neighbor again and discuss what they learned from this assessment. (5 minutes)

6) The trainer reconvenes the group and solicits observations from participants. After several comments and illustrations have been shared, she offers a final thought on enhancing self-esteem.

● Any self-change—even desirable change—usually meets resistance. Just as our body's homeostatic mechanism seeks to keep our temperature constant, our psyche strives to maintain the status quo. Familiar patterns seem safer than new ones—even when there is potential for positive payoff.

● **Building self-esteem is a lifetime agenda that requires vigilance and persistence**. You may not notice changes immediately, but when you look back from a distance, you will recognize that your daily efforts at viewing yourself more positively have made a big difference in your life.

VARIATIONS

■ The planning process, *Discoveries* (p 100), and the closing ritual, *Whisper Circle* (p 111), would fit well with this exercise. Affirming energizers such as *Megaphone* (**Wellness 1**), *Cheers!* (**Wellness 2**) and *Get Off My Back* (**Stress 1**) could be inserted between *Steps 3* and *4*. For another approach to self-esteem, check out *The Fourth Source of Stress* (**Stress 2**).

■ With a large group (50–100 people), pair up participants and give each pair a card with one characteristic of high or low self-esteem from the grid. Participants discuss how this trait enhances (or deflates) self-esteem. After 2–3 minutes of discussion the trainer asks for reports from the pairs and weaves their answers into a series of mini-lectures on various aspects of self-esteem. Participants can take the whole test on the spot or save it for homework.

Submitted by Krysta Eryn Kavenaugh.

CHARACTERISTICS OF *LOW* SELF-ESTEEM

	A	B	C
1. feel and act like a "victim"			
2. judgmental of self and others			
3. break agreements, violate own standards			
4. covert, phony			
5. exaggerate, pretend, lie			
6. self-deprecating, shameful, blaming, critical, condemning			
7. "nice" person, approval-seeking, people pleaser			
8. negative attitude			
9. rationalize			
10. jealous/envious of others			
11. perfectionist			
12. dependencies, addictions; compulsive, self-destructive			
13. complacent, stagnant			
14. not liking the work one does			
15. leave tasks and relationships unfinished			
16. judge self-worth by comparing to others; feel inferior			
17. don't accept or give compliments			
18. excessive worry			
19. fearful of exploring "real self"			
20. shun new endeavors, fearing mistakes or failure			
21. irrational responses, ruled by emotions			
22. lack of purpose in life			
23. feel inadequate to handle new situations			
24. feel resentful and "one down" when I lose			
25. vulnerable to others' opinion, comments, attitudes			

D.

E. I've learned . . .

CHARACTERISTICS OF *HIGH* SELF-ESTEEM

	F	G	H
1. take appropriate risks			
2. take responsibility for life and consequences of actions			
3. have life purpose, goal-directed, committed			
4. honest with self and others emotionally and intellectually			
5. face and move through fears			
6. admit mistakes, shortcomings, defeats; accept limitations			
7. develop strengths; respect, nourish, accept, trust self			
8. do own thinking and make own decisions			
9. forgiving of self and others			
10. tenacity/persistence			
11. attitude of gratitude			
12. accepting of self and others			
13. set and follow internal standards/principles/values;			
14. see opportunities instead of problems			
15. positive attitude, zest, enthusiastic, spontaneous			
16. praise self and others			
17. see the big picture; continual striving for growth			
18. can appropriately ask for help			
19. anticipate new endeavors with quiet confidence			
20. actively participate in life			
21. on ooccasion enjoy being alone			
22. "to thine own self be true"			
23. allow self to be human/make mistakes			
24. share real self			
25. aim for excellence, not perfection			

J.

_____

K. I've learned . . .

©1994 Whole Person Press 210 W Michigan Duluth MN 55802   (800) 247-6789

124 WELLNESS MEDITATION

The cleansing breaths of this affirming visualization allow participants to find inner harmony and peace.

GOALS

To practice a health-enhancing centering and relaxation experience.

To reinforce the mind/body/spirit connection in well-being.

GROUP SIZE

Unlimited.

TIME FRAME

15 minutes

MATERIALS NEEDED

Wellness Meditation script; tape recorder and relaxing music.

PROCESS

☞ *This exercise is especially effective just before a break or at the close of a meeting. Leave the music playing for several minutes after the end of the meditation, allowing people to luxuriate in their peaceful feelings.*

1) The trainer introduces the exercise with a few comments on health and wholeness.

   ● The goal of wellness is to experience your body, mind and spirit interacting in a harmony that promotes wholeness and well-being.

   ● A balanced diet, regular exercise, effective stress management and other healthy lifestyle decisions contribute to this whole person well-being.

   ● We can heighten our experience of the synergy of the whole by engaging in regular centering meditation that draws the body/mind/spirit threads of life together and sharpens our inner awareness of peace and well-being.

2) The trainer turns on background music and invites participants to sit back, close their eyes, relax as much as possible and prepare for a

peaceful, healing journey. As soon as the group settles down, he reads the **Wellness Meditation** script.

☞ *Read slowly and expressively. Allow plenty of time for participants to form the images and enjoy the sensations.*

3) If the meditation is not followed by a break, the trainer may solicit a few reactions from participants before moving on to the next content segment.

WELLNESS MEDITATION Script

Allow yourself to relax as much as possible in your chair . . .
with your hands resting comfortably in your lap . . . .
Uncross your legs and let your feet be flat on the floor . . . .
Take in a deep breath . . .
and as you exhale . . . let your eyes close . . . .
Continue to take slow . . . deep . . . easy breaths . . . .

Think of each breath as cleansing you . . .
clean fresh air coming in like a cool drink . . . .
And each time you exhale . . .
let your tensions flow with the current of air out of your body . . . .
Think only about your breathing . . .
and let anything else on your mind flow out with your breath . . . .
Feel yourself relaxing . . .
as each breath removes the tensions and worries of your day . . . .

Feel the weight of your hands in your lap . . .
and imagine them floating as if on clouds . . . .
There is no tension in your arms . . .
as they are floating lightly with your hands . . . .
Your shoulders settle down as your muscles relax . . .
and your head may drop slightly down and forward . . . .
With each breath, you become even more relaxed and at ease . . . .

You may become aware of your heart beating smoothly and
rhythmically . . . .
You can feel the blood pulsing through your body . . .
to your legs and feet . . . to your arms and fingers . . .
flowing to every cell . . . bringing the oxygen of your breath . . . .
Feel each breath flowing deeply into your body . . .
bringing life to every part . . . .

The blood also carries the nutrients from your last meal . . . .
What you have eaten has been absorbed . . .
and now this nourishment flows to rebuild and strengthen your body . . . .
Energy is delivered to every cell and stored for ready use . . . .

Imagine your body using that energy . . .
moving with ease and grace . . . .
Think back to a time when you enjoyed some playful movement . . .
carefree and fun . . . .
Remember the buoyant feeling of freedom . . . *and how good you felt* . . . .

Continue to ride these feelings . . . *moving freely* . . .
and passing through time to another place . . .
a favorite place where you feel safe, calm and contented . . . .
It may be a garden or a meadow . . .
a secluded shore or under the brilliant night sky . . .
wherever is your favorite place . . . .

You can feel the peace and tranquillity of this special place . . . .
You feel like you belong here . . . .
You are at peace with yourself and your world . . . .

And as you think of the beauty and specialness of your favorite place . . .
you realize the miracle of its creation . . . *and your own* . . . .
There is peace within you now . . .
as you tune in to yourself and your Creator . . .
knowing the joy of this life-giving connection . . . .

Now it's time to start coming back to this room . . .
to the present place and time . . . .
But you can bring the peace with you . . .
and make it an ever-present part of your life . . . .
As you nurture yourself and others with wholesome food . . .
as you enjoy the spirit of play . . .
as you experience the acceptance of one another . . .
and the love of the Creator . . . *this peace will remain with you* . . . .

And if you should lose this feeling of peace . . .
you know you can come back and find it any time . . .
just the way you did here . . . *for it is always present within you* . . . .

Open your eyes when you are ready . . . *and go in peace* . . . .

Submitted by Grant Christopher.

125 EXPANDING YOUR CIRCLES

Participants explore preconceived notions about who belongs in their "inner circle" and experiment with attitude changes that can build a wider support system.

GOALS

To demonstrate that our attitude, not the worth of other people, determines who we will exclude from our lives and who we will include.

To encourage the development of a broader, more varied support network through attitude readjustment.

GROUP SIZE

Unlimited.

TIME FRAME

20–30 minutes

PROCESS

1) The trainer notes that healthy, supportive relationships contribute significantly to our sense of well-being. He invites participants to consider their friendship and support networks and offers some opening comments on how people develop "circles" of friends.

   ● It is common to mentally sort people we know into a variety of categories. We don't necessarily label each person. Rather, we "draw" vague circles in our minds about where people fit, based on how trustworthy we feel they are, how close we feel to them, how committed we are to them, etc.

   ● Our innermost circle includes only a few people—our most trusted family and best friends. The next circle we may call friends and the next circle acquaintances. As we move further and further from our inner circle, our trust level and commitment to the people "out there" diminishes. Eventually the circles end and we consider all those people outside our widest circle as strangers.

   ● Although this sorting of people into the "circles we move in" is a natural process, based on our preconceived expectations and our personal history, most of our judgments about who belongs where are based on very little information. This is especially true for those we place in the outer fringes. We write off whole groups of people and exclude them from our potential "neighborhood"—without ever really knowing who they are.

2) The trainer invites participants to explore their support systems by drawing the circles of their neighborhood.

> ☞ *Allow ample time for participants to complete each instruction before reading the next.*

➤ Take a blank sheet of paper and start by drawing a small circle in the middle to represent your *self.*

➤ Next, draw a bigger circle around *self* for your *family and intimate friends.* List by name each person who belongs in this "tender" circle.

➤ Now make a larger circle for those people you would identify as *friends.* As you list your friends, don't forget to include the special people on your Christmas card list!

➤ Next, draw a still larger circle to include all your *acquaintances that you know by name.* List neighbors, work associates, service people, church members, etc.

➤ Now draw a still bigger circle for acquaintances whom you recognize, but *whose names you don't know.* Use symbols to represent neighbors, work associates, service people, church members, etc that you know only by sight.

➤ Finally, *outside your circle* at the edge of the paper, list all the types of people that you automatically exclude from your circle of relationships. Perhaps those who are handicapped or of a different skin color. Maybe people who are much older or much younger than you. Perhaps odd, fragile, disoriented, dirty or tattered people. Maybe very rich people or people from another part of the country or those who lack manners or speak with poor grammar. Or, perhaps powerful executives or evangelists or secular humanists.

Be honest with yourself and list whatever kinds of people you shy away from because they make you feel uncomfortable in some way. List all these folks at the edge of your paper, outside your circle.

3) The trainer invites participants to consider the power of personal attitudes in the process of developing relationships and deciding who will be part of our support system circles.

- **Our attitudes to a great extent determine which people we will let into our circles.** The tighter we draw our circles, the more we close ourselves off from a world full of neighbors.

- If we develop the attitude that every person has something unique to offer us, we can begin to expand the *circles we run in*—and fill our lives with more varied and stimulating relationships.

- **Our challenge then becomes to unlock and discover the potential beauty in each person.** If we open our eyes and mind, and perk up our ears, we are more likely to experience the best of what each person can offer us—and we will enrich our own lives by the experience.

4) The trainer asks participants to examine their *circles* worksheet and to consider changing their attitudes toward some of the people listed on their sheets.

➤ Choose one person from each of your relationship circles (and one person from those outside your circle) whom you would consider moving inward one circle (eg, making an *undesirable* an *acquaintance*, or a *face* into a *name*, or a *name* into a *friend*, or a *friend* into an *intimate*).

➤ Highlight the person you select in each circle.

➤ Now consider each person whom you have chosen to move one circle closer to you. Think about these people. Wonder about their uniqueness. Ask yourself:

    ➤ What needs might they have?
    ➤ What is their story? Their history?
    ➤ What pain have they known?
    ➤ What are their interests? Skills? Worries?
    ➤ What might be their beauty?

➤ Consider what *you* could do to reach out to each of these people and to move them into a circle closer to you. How could you move them one step closer?

➤ Jot down your ideas for each person. Then, at your next contact, DO IT! And enjoy what happens!

5) The trainer divides participants into small discussion groups and invites them to share their observations on the circles they have drawn and the attitudes that created these circles, as well as their resolutions for who and how to move a few people one circle closer. (10–15 minutes)

6) The trainer regathers the entire group and solicits feedback on their observations and insights. He concludes the exercise by offering participants the following suggestions for widening the circles of their support network and thus enriching their lives.

- **Develop the willingness to risk**. It's easier to reach out to those who are the closest, and harder to reach out to those in the outer circles. Work on your fear. Practice walking across the room and opening a conversation in as many different ways as you can each day. You'll get used to it!

- **Prepare to give of yourself**. Reach out and touch people with your eyes and ears, with your questions and your interest in them. It won't always work out, but overall you will be rewarded in surprising ways.

- **Develop a tolerance for difference**. Not everyone is just like you—thank God! Wouldn't that be boring! As you mature and open yourself you can learn to tolerate, even appreciate, a greater variety of differences in the people around you.

- **Focus on the positive**. Practice being curious and expectant rather than afraid or judgmental. Look for the beauty of the other person to unfold as you show interest in them. And if that doesn't happen every time, don't worry. It doesn't prove anything. Just try again.

TRAINER'S NOTES

126 DEPTH FINDER

Participants use a checklist to explore their values, then develop a graphic representation of their personal value systems.

GOALS

To reinforce the importance of values as sources of life meaning and shapers of health choices.

To examine value system components and clarify values that are personally significant.

GROUP SIZE

Unlimited, as long as there are plenty of art supplies and table space for making graphic designs.

TIME FRAME

30–45 minutes

MATERIALS NEEDED

Depth Finder worksheets and blank paper for all; a wide variety of assorted crayons, markers and colored pencils within easy reach of each participant.

PROCESS

1) The trainer begins with an introductory chalktalk on the nature, function and importance of values.

   ● **The search for meaning and meaningful values is a basic motivating force for human beings**. We yearn for a "center" around which to develop a meaningful life—a core to provide vision and a direction for growth. We search for guiding principles that help us distinguish right and wrong, that provide a framework for making choices.

   ● The values that hold us together and provide this internal guidance include our *personal preferences* (feeling-based), our *morals* (conscience-based "shoulds" and "should-nots"), our *beliefs* (leaps of faith without proof) and our *actions* through which we integrate and implement the other three.

- **Values shape our decisions and choices in all areas of life—including health and self-care.** Values help us decide how to use our resources (time, energy, environment, relationships, dollars) most constructively.

- **An unexamined value system may trap us in unhealthy patterns.** Conflicting values can immobilize us. If we make a conscious effort to clarify our values, and allow our value system to remain open to new information, values can be a powerful health promotion resource.

2) The trainer announces that participants will have an opportunity to examine some aspects of their value system—using both sides of their brains. He distributes **Depth Finder** worksheets to everyone and gives step-by-step instructions for completing them.

   ➤ This instrument is designed to help you identify the major values that characterize your life. In each section of the worksheet (*orientation, expression, life goals, value shapers*), circle words that describe qualities or values that strongly influence your choices in life.

   The circled items may have either *good* or *bad* connotations for you. The issue is the strength of their influence on you. Feel free to add any other significant items if key values are missing.

   ☞ *Remind people that this is an instrument for self-awareness, not a character reference! So they can be fully honest in their responses. Allow 3–5 minutes, then move on to the next step.*

   ➤ Look over the *Values Shapers* section of the worksheet and identify with a *star* the five items that are *most important to you.* (1 minute)

   ➤ Now look over the *Values Shapers* list again, and pick out five personal desires that you would most like to *improve or change.* (1 minute)

   ➤ Mentally step back and take a look at the big picture. Examine all the words you have circled and notice any major incongruity or conflicts among the values. If you see any potential discordances, make some notes about your observations at the bottom of the worksheet.

   ➤ As a final step, connect all the words you circled with a line so you can see your values map.

3) The trainer distributes blank paper and drawing utensils to participants and invites them to try another approach to values exploration—this time using their right brain functions of intuition, creativity and seeing overall patterns.

➤ Use crayons, colored pencils, markers or a mixture of all three to create a graphic design that represents the different components and expressions of your value system, including preferences, desires, moral values, goals, beliefs and actions.

➤ You may want to consult your **Depth Finder** assessment and incorporate whatever strikes you in your graphic design (eg, if you identified conflicts in your values you might want to portray these graphically or you may want to focus on your five key values).

Feel free to include words or labels in your design. Let the colors and shapes express your feelings and insights.

🖝 *Remind people they don't have to be artists. Encourage reluctant participants to choose a color and start doodling— something is bound to take shape. Allow 5–8 minutes for the drawing.*

➤ Now look at your finished design and write down your reactions to what you see. (1 minute)

4) The trainer notes that one criterion of a value is that we must be willing to publicly affirm it. She instructs participants to form groups of four (or rejoin small groups) for a time of affirming values.

➤ Take turns sharing some aspect of your value system with the others in your group.

➤ As a starting point, you may want to show your graphic design to the group and describe what you see or what it means. Or you may want to talk about insights you gained in completing your **Depth Finder** assessment.

➤ Each person should take 2–3 minutes to talk about your values. I'll let you know when the time is about half gone so you can pace yourselves and make sure everyone gets a chance to share.

5) The trainer interrupts after 5–7 minutes to give the halftime signal. When everyone has had a chance to share (10–15 minutes) the trainer reconvenes the large group and solicits summary insights, observations and reactions from participants.

The Depth Finder assessment and process was submitted by Larry Chapman. The values system graphic design was adapted from an idea in Lucia Capacchione's **Creative Journal** *(Athens OH: Ohio University Press).*

DEPTH FINDER

My Basic Orientation	Idea-Centered		God-Centered	Person-Centered
Major Life Goals	Wealth Status Fulfillment Growth	Love Power Truth Knowledge	Security Peace Excellence Comfort	Self-Acceptance Achievement Contribution Relationships
Values Shapers	Commitment Experience Excitement Decency Actualization Serving Others Affection Unmarried Control Independence Travel Kindness Superiority Alcohol Isolation Self-Sacrifice Happiness Rejection Sexual Lack Aloof Self-Serving Gregarious Resisting Change Negative Strength Acceptance Beauty Shy Adventure Affluence		Self-Discipline Marriage Leisure Sexual Pleasure Friendship Anger Meaning Honesty Revenge Challenge Assertiveness Advantage Accountability Freedom Dishonesty Pain-Seeking Drug-Free Pleasure Justice Vulnerable Resentful Playful Quiet Insecure Competence Ease Curiosity Unfaithful Self-Confidence Ritual	Pain-Avoidance Integrity Cooperation Kindness Cheerfulness Education Instant Gratification Wellness Children Position Sloth Self-Importance Goodness Irresponsibility Job Satisfaction Intimacy Selfishness Detachment Openness Rebellious Fitness Forgiveness Accepting Change Compulsiveness Criticism Illness Hatred Equality Respect Conflict

127 LET'S PLAY

Participants explore the health-enhancing benefits of play in this light-hearted look at a serious subject.

GOALS

To examine personal play quotients and styles.

To rediscover the importance of play in a healthy lifestyle.

To uncover barriers to play.

GROUP SIZE

Described for 20–40 people; adaptable for larger groups.

TIME FRAME

40–45 minutes

MATERIALS NEEDED

Blackboard or newsprint easel.

PROCESS

☞ *This exercise makes an excellent companion to a presentation on Type A behavior or the health risks of the workaholic pattern (see* **Lifetrap 1: Workaholism, Stress 1** *and* **Lifetrap 2: Hooked on Helping, Stress 2**).

1) The trainer begins by announcing that the group will be considering a serious health issue—play! He solicits from the group examples of words they associate with play (eg, fun, games, spontaneity, childlike, etc).

   ☞ *To model the concept that play is possible under almost any conditions, affirm all the ideas that are generated. You may want to record the suggestions on newsprint.*

2) The trainer makes a brief presentation on the nature of play, using examples participants have generated to illustrate some or all of the following points.

   ● **Play is a natural, healthy function for all animals**—even adult human beings! Play can involve us in exploration, role rehearsal, social interaction, creativity, emotional expression, cognitive development, values clarification, and skill practice—all while we're having fun! As children we learn and grow through play. As adults we continue the process.

- **Play is re-creation.** Play is a special kind of self-nurture that revitalizes and refreshes the body/mind/spirit.
- When we go for long periods without play, we lose spirit and vitality. All work and no play makes Jack a prime candidate for a heart attack!
- **Play is also rebellious.** When we play we often break the conventional cause-and-effect rules of our otherwise ordered lives. The spontaneity, imagination and emotional involvement that characterize play temporarily free us for improvisation and experimentation without worrying about the outcome.
- **Play is an essential component for intimacy in relationships.** People who play together stay together—when they use their playfulness to handle conflicts, alter moods and nurture their "culture of two."

3) In preparation for the next activity, the trainer asks someone in the group to name an animal. When someone suggests an animal, the trainer asks the person to demonstrate the sound that the animal makes. He then leads participants in a group rendition of the animal sound.

> ☞ *Ham this up a bit. Start with soft noises, then repeat several times getting louder and louder. You may want to throw in some appropriate actions to fit the animal. Remind people that this is an exercise in PLAY!*

4) The trainer solicits two more suggestions of animals from the group, and repeats the group "chorus" with each.

> ☞ *After the third animal's sounds are completed, run the group quickly back through the three choruses again.*

5) The trainer invites participants to join in a playful fantasy and reads the **Meadow Frolic** script, p. 81.

> ☞ *For clarity, three animals are named in the script (a cow, cat and monkey). When you read the script, substitute the three animals chosen by your group.*

MEADOW FROLIC Script

Close your eyes for a moment . . . take a deep breath . . . and relax as
comfortably as you can . . . .

Let an image of a grassy meadow begin to form in your mind . . . a lovely
meadow where the sun is shining and the air is pleasantly warm . . . .

Let the meadow take shape in your mind . . . .
Perhaps there are trees for shade . . . with deep grass . . . or a brook
running through the meadow . . . or a fence by the road . . . maybe a
building in the distance . . . .

Now you notice that there are three animals frolicking in the
meadow . . . (a cow) . . . and (a cat) . . . and (a monkey) . . . .

☞ *Remember to insert your group's animals.*

You stop and watch them play . . .
and notice how each animal enjoys the freedom and fun of their play . . . .

Continue to watch all the different ways these animals play together in the
fresh clean air and warm sunshine . . . .

☞ *Pause here for 30 seconds or more so participants can*
"play" with this fantasy. You might want to try it yourself!

After a time you notice that the sun is beginning to slide toward the
horizon . . . and one of the animals leaves the meadow . . . .
You watch the animal move away . . . and then return your attention to the
other two animals who are sill playing joyously in the meadow . . . .

You watch their antics for a while longer . . .
until the sun sinks deeper and the shadows grow longer . . .
and one of the remaining two animals leaves the scene . . . .

One animal is left in the meadow . . . playing alone . . .
enjoying the cool breeze and the fading light . . . .

And now you turn and leave the meadow . . .
and slowly return to this room . . .
looking back occasionally to see the solitary animal still playing in the
meadow . . . .

And when you're ready to leave the fantasy behind . . .
and rejoin us in this room . . . open your eyes . . . .

6) The trainer announces that the next activity requires that participants move to an open space in the room and form three groups. He then gives instructions for the process.

➤ Please stand up. Recall the last animal that was playing in your imaginary meadow.

➤ When I give the signal, start making the sound of that animal, and then move to the open area where you should search out and gather with the other animals of your kind, joining voices in a loud chorus. GO!

7) When the three groups are formed and vocalizing, the trainer interrupts the cacophony with instructions for the next step.

➤ Everyone close one eye. Now pair up with someone in your animal group who has closed the same eye.

☞ *If there are odd numbers, pair up the leftovers from two groups and/or take the extra person as your partner.*

➤ Decide who is **Monopoly** and who is **Scrabble.**

➤ The **Scrabble** partner will begin. Take 3 minutes to describe all the ways you can remember playing as a child. The **Monopoly** partners should listen closely and show your interest **non-verbally.**

➤ I'll let you know when 3 minutes are up so that you can switch roles.

8) The trainer interrupts after 3 minutes and directs the **Monopoly** partner to share childhood play activities. After 3 minutes he interrupts again and asks participants to return to their seats. When everyone is settled, the trainer solicits observations and insights from the group.

☞ *The energy level of the group is usually charged up by this exchange, as people recall all the playfulness of childhood and begin to wonder what's happened to their play quotient as adults. Use comments of this nature to make a transition to the brainstorming in the next step.*

9) The trainer notes that participants seem to know more about play than they expected! He asks the group to identify some of their **personal barriers to play**—thoughts and reservations that keep them from playing more (eg, guilt, work comes first, family rules, don't want to appear foolish, not productive, feel vulnerable, etc). All barriers mentioned by the group are listed on the chalkboard or newsprint.

☞ *After the group has generated a substantial list, encourage people to dig behind the obvious barriers to some of their more personal, private, unspoken (even unconscious) barriers (eg, power/control issues, fear of intimacy, role conflicts, not deserving happiness, shame, etc).*

10) Next the trainer challenges the group to come up with a list of **benefits to play** that is at least as long as the list of barriers. As participants brainstorm benefits, the trainer lists them on the board and elaborates as necessary to highlight the following points.

● **Play is a valuable and mature activity**—even in public. Play can help us change our mood and alter our perspective. Even as adults we develop and practice vital lifeskills through play, including laughter, humor, fantasy, spontaneity, trust and acceptance.

● **Play is an attitude as well as an activity**. Playfulness can often transform the "required" into the "desired." In fact, play is a healthy antidote to stress and can counteract the seriousness that permeates the rest of our life.

11) The trainer asks for a show of hands on two questions.

✔ How many people imagine that they will feel guilty if they take more time for play?

☞ *For those brave souls who say "yes," announce that you have just what they need. Draw a large prescription form on the board. Put an "Rx" at the top and then write the notation "PLAY q.i.d." (four times a day) or "PLAY p.r.n." (as needed). Then sign your name (Dr. So-and-So) with a flourish, and tell participants, "Now you can tell anyone who asks that the doctor told you to play!"*

✔ How many people would like to put a little more play in their life?

☞ *Congratulate these "converts" to play—and then playfully suggest that the others must have missed the point and will need a remedial class in play. Then proceed to the final step.*

12) The trainer invites participants to construct their personal fun house of potential play activities that they can use as a prompt for putting more play in their life.

➤ Take out a blank sheet of paper and draw a large house. This is your fun house.

➤ Based on what you've remembered today about yourself and your natural playfulness, spend a couple of minutes **listing inside your fun house all the activities that you enjoy doing** (eg, shopping, playing golf, dancing, gambling, movies, sex, reading to your kids, gardening, pillow fights, making funny noises, etc). Don't forget the outrageous, silly, playful, child-like ways to have fun.

➤ If you get stuck, jog your memory by thinking through your day yesterday, or the last few weekends, or the cycle of the seasons. Also remember what you've learned about play from other people in this sesison.

☞ *Allow at least 5 minutes for this process. If people get restless, encourage them to write a detailed plan for exactly when, where and what they will do to play in the next 24 or 48 hours.*

13) The trainer challenges participants to add another item to their fun house.

➤ Think of some activity you must do frequently, even though you don't enjoy doing it (eg, washing dishes, finishing paper work at the office, cooking, balancing the checkbook, riding the bus, attending committee meetings, etc). Consider how you might make this activity more fun—*play* around with ideas for adding a playful dimension to this mundane activity.

14) The trainer solicits examples of playful agendas that people have planned and then leads the group in a playful closing energizer (eg, *Joke Around,* p 123).

VARIATIONS

■ *Humorous Interludes (**Stress 1**), Month of Fundays (**Stress 2**)* and *The Garden* reading (***Stress 2***) would make excellent additions to this process. To help the group indulge in some additional on-the-spot playfulness, try the energizers *Clapdance* (p 118), *Microwave* (***Stress 4***), *Groans and Moans (**Stress 3**), Red Rover (**Wellness 1**)* or *Outrageous Episodes (**Wellness 3**).*

■ Duplicate some special "Prescriptions for Play" and distribute them to all participants as part of *Step 11.*

*Submitted by Michael Metz who adapted some of the process from Weinstein and Goodman's classic on the subject, **Playfair** (Impact Publishers, 1980).*

128 JOB MOTIVATORS

In this examination of needs and motivation, participants determine their personal priorities for job satisfaction and assess the degree to which their current life work fulfills their top-ranked needs.

GOALS

To examine the multi-faceted reasons for working.

To assess the degree to which one's current job fulfills major work-related needs.

GROUP SIZE

Unlimited.

TIME FRAME

40–50 minutes

MATERIALS NEEDED

Blackboard or flip chart; **Job Motivators Inventory** worksheets.

PROCESS

1) The trainer introduces the exercise by asking the group for some examples of why people work, then weaves the participants' responses into a chalktalk on personal needs, job satisfaction and well-being.

  - **Jobs provide a complex mixture of rewards**. There are many reasons for working. Although nearly everyone is motivated in part by the rewards of the "employee benefit package" (wages, insurance, pension, vacation, etc), there are many other human needs that can be fulfilled by our work. In this session we are going to look at a dozen job motivators that usually don't show up in the contract but are as important to most workers as their salaries.

  - **Each of us wants something different from our work**. Your personal job satisfaction hierarchy is as unique as your fingerprint— and for most people nearly as unexamined and unfamiliar.

  - **No one job can ever meet all our needs**. But for a job to be fulfilling, it must meet some of the basic needs that you consider essential. When a job doesn't satisfy some of your key needs, it drains you rather than energizing you.

- **What you want out of your job may change.** As you grow as a person, as you gain confidence or competence, as your life situation shifts, as the nature of your work changes, you may find different needs taking priority—and you may discover that your job has become more or less satisfying than before.
- Since most of us spend a large part of the day working, **on-the-job satisfaction can contribute significantly to our over-all sense of well-being.** During this exercise we will examine a variety of qualities in the work environment that may motivate you to perform effectively and make your job fulfilling.

2) The trainer distributes **Job Motivation Inventory** worksheets and gives instructions for the first assessment. (3–5 minutes)

➤ Look over the list of 12 job motivators. For each category, ask yourself the question, *"Do I work for this reason?"*

➤ Use a 1 to 3 scale to rate your response, and record the number for each motivator in *Column A.*

   1 = Not Really.
   2 = A Little Bit/Sometimes/Somewhat.
   3 = Absolutely! This is a primary motivator for me.

3) The trainer instructs participants to pair up with a neighbor and compare notes on their top and bottom job motivators. If there is time, partners discuss why they have made these needs top (or bottom) priority at this point in their lives. (3–5 minutes)

4) The trainer interrupts the pairs and gives instructions for the next part of the *Inventory.*

➤ Consider each category of job motivators again. This time rate how well this need is fulfilled by your *current job.* Write your response to the question, *"Is this need met in my present work?"* in *Column B,* using the following scale:

   1 = No, not really.
   2 = Somewhat.
   3 = Yes, to a large extent.

➤ As you mark your rating, make some notes to yourself in *Column C* about the ways your needs are (or are not) met. What improvements would you like to see?

5) As most participants finish up this task, the trainer directs them to compare the two rankings they have recorded for each of the 12

categories (*Column A:* Important to me? *Column B:* Fulfilled in present job?).

☞ *You may want to point out that most stress occurs in categories where the fulfillment of a need and its ranking as a priority are at variance. If a need is rated "absolutely essential" as a motivator, but is not being fulfilled on the job, frustration will increase. Little stress results, however when a need that is left unfulfilled by the job is also ranked as "not really important."*

6) The trainer invites participants to reflect in more depth on their overall job satisfaction and its relationship to personal needs by answering *Questions 1* to *5* on the *Reflection* section of the worksheet. (5 minutes)

☞ *You may want to guide the group through this process to keep everyone moving at about the same pace, and to clarify any ambiguities.*

7) The trainer divides participants into groups of 4–6 persons each, or reconvenes previous small groups and gives instructions for sharing.

➤ Spend 3–4 minutes each sharing the insights you gained from filling out your worksheets.

    ➤ Each person should begin by reading your list of priority needs (*Question # 1*)—those items a job absolutely must fulfill for you.

    ➤ Then read your description of the perfect job and what it would give you (*Question # 2*).

    ➤ Finally, take some time to tell the others in your group how your current job does—or does not—meet these needs.

☞ *Encourage participants to listen carefully to each other and to mentally note areas of similarity and difference in the personal need priorities expressed.*

8) The trainer reconvenes the total group and solicits observations and insights from the small group discussions.

9) The trainer notes that there are five options for increasing the degree to which job-related needs are being met. As she outlines the five alternatives, participants are invited to consider how these options might apply to their own life/work situations.

☞ *Write each option on the blackboard or newsprint as you go along so that participants can refer to them in the next step.*

- **Alter your job so that it fulfills more of your needs.** This may not be easy, and you may not have total control, but often you can make small changes (sometimes without anyone else even noticing) that will significantly enhance your job satisfaction.

- **Look for fulfillment of some unmet job needs through your personal life.** Too much of this strategy might be dangerous, but sometimes you can take the edge off your frustration on the job by getting some of your needs met outside the work setting. For example, if relationships in your work environment are characterized by conflict, make sure that you build supportive friendships outside your work world.

- **Find fulfillment of unmet job needs through volunteer work.** If your job doesn't give you all that you want, tackle a position in the community that will. For example, if your daily work isn't challenging enough, volunteer for a task that is. Or if your job doesn't allow for much creativity, find a community project that requires dreaming.

- **Decide that you're getting enough satisfaction from your job right now!** Accept it as it is. No job is perfect. Don't spend your life grumbling about minor irritants in your job if it is, in fact, giving you a large measure of fulfillment.

- **Look for another job that will be more fulfilling and rewarding for you.** Yes, if you've discovered during this reflection process that your job is simply not fulfilling enough of your needs, a career change may be in order. You might want to start looking for something else that will be more motivating. You can't just thumb your nose at the security you have in your current job, but you do have the right to expect a lot more than just money when you invest yourself in your work.

10) The trainer instructs participants to consider which option seems to hold the most promise for increasing their level of job satisfaction. In closing, people make some notes about the specific steps they plan to take.

VARIATIONS

■ To add an intriguing icebreaker to this exercise, use the **Job Motivators** list in combination with *Wheel of Fortune, p 11*. Participants discuss a different job motivator with each partner, sharing where—or if—that item has been motivating for them.

■ Instead of using the 12 categories outlined on the worksheet, let the group generate their own list of job motivators as part of *Step 1*. This list would be substituted for that on the worksheets as participants examine their personal needs (*Steps 2* to *5*). The rest of the exercise would continue as described.

TRAINER'S NOTES

JOB MOTIVATORS INVENTORY

Circle those items in each category that most apply to you.
Cross out those items that don't apply to you at all.

	A	B	C

1. Employment Package
■ To have enough money for
    my lifestyle
    my family
    my future
■ To get ahead financially
■ To be safe and insured for
    unexpected emergencies
    or crises			

2. Variety
■ To have a change of pace from
    my personal and home life
■ To have balanced and reasonable
    hours and schedule
■ To experience true separation
    between work and home			

3. Positive Environment
■ To have a pleasant work environ-
    ment, conducive to physical/
    mental health
■ To be located in a desirable area
■ To experience beauty			

4. Sense of Worth ■ To feel good about myself ■ To experience confidence and personal power			
5. Affirmation ■ To receive recognition for my work ■ To be seen as highly skilled ■ To be looked up to with respect			

6. Relationships
■ To meet a variety of new people
■ To be accepted
■ To feel care from others and for
    them as well
■ To experience camaraderie and a
    sense of belonging			

JOB MOTIVATORS INVENTORY

Circle those items in each category that most apply to you.
Cross out those items that don't apply to you at all.

	A	B	C
7. Connection ■ To experience being part of a team ■ To be part of an organization of which I am proud ■ To know I am an important part of the whole			
8. Control ■ To have freedom to organize my work as I see best ■ To be responsible for specific decisions			
9. Productivity ■ To have an opportunity to be creative: to make something to make up something to make something happen ■ To accomplish something, be productive ■ To solve problems			
10. Stimulation ■ To add excitement and adventure ■ To push me to grow and advance ■ To develop myself and my skills			
11. Usefulness ■ To use my talents effectively ■ To match well with my interests, skills and abilities			
12. Purpose ■ To give meaning to my life ■ To help others and make the world a better place ■ To grow in depth and understanding of the world and my place in it			

©1994 Whole Person Press 210 W Michigan Duluth MN 55802   (800) 247-6789

JOB MOTIVATORS: REFLECTION

1) List your top priority needs that a job must meet for you—those conditions that are absolutely essential to keep you motivated.

   At a minimum I must have:

   1.   *2.*

   3.   *4.*

2) Describe the perfect job situation for you by completing the following paragraph. (Don't exaggerate—be realistic. But **do** express what *you want* out of a job.)

   My perfect job would give me . . .

3) On a scale of 1 to 10 rank your current job against the standards of your "perfect"job.

   1 = My current job gives me nothing I want;
   10 = I'm totally fulfilled in my current job

   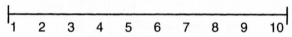

   1   2   3   4   5   6   7   8   9   10

4) Comment on the extent to which your highest priority needs are—or are not— being met by your present job:

5) How has the fulfillment—or lack of fulfillment of these key needs affected your sense of vocational well-being and current job-related satisfaction?

129 INFORMATION IS NOT ENOUGH

In this reflection process participants explore their beliefs about a personal health problem and discover how they can turn information and good intentions into appropriate action.

GOALS

To recognize the power of beliefs and perceptions as motivators or barriers to action.

To promote health-enhancing behaviors and increase self-care follow through.

GROUP SIZE

Unlimited.

TIME FRAME

20–30 minutes

MATERIALS NEEDED

Blank paper for all.

PROCESS

1) The trainer begins by asking participants to respond to three questions:

   ✔ Has anyone ever neglected good self-care, or ever indulged in some harmful behavior, even though you knew better (eg, smoking, poor eating habits, high stress, etc)?

   ☞ *Acknowledge that people are in good company, that no one is perfect! For this and the next two questions, ask for examples and comments on why people don't take better care of themselves.*

   ✔ Have you ever ignored symptoms that might indicate a potential health problem?

   ✔ Has anyone ever failed to follow through on a treatment plan recommended by a doctor, nurse, dentist, counselor, dietitian, physical therapist, etc?

2) The trainer weaves examples solicited from the group in *Step 1* into a brief summary of research on the relationship between information and self-care practices.

- During the 1950's researchers studying people attending tuberculosis screening clinics discovered that information was not the sole, or even the primary, factor determining whether or not people would follow through with prevention and treatment plans.
- Instead, **people's behavior was influenced by their** *beliefs*—their perceptions of the severity of the disease, their assumptions about how susceptible they were personally and their beliefs about the potential drawbacks and benefits of the recommended action.
- Subsequent research on other preventive health behaviors such as Pap smears, immunizations, and blood pressure screenings confirms these earlier findings that **beliefs and perceptions—not information—are the keys to self-care action.**

3) The trainer distributes blank paper and invites participants to apply the health belief model to a personal health concern.

➤ First, *identify a current personal health concern* where you have not taken appropriate action.

   ➤ This concern could be some way in which you have wanted to *take better care of yourself* (eg, STOP smoking, eating desserts, worrying so much; START relaxing more, exercising, developing wider support networks, etc).

   ➤ Or this concern could be a *symptom that is bothering you;* a symptom that you should pay attention to or seek consultation for (eg, alcohol use, back pain, depression, headaches, lack of meaning, sense of isolation, overworking, difficulty making decisions, etc).

   ➤ Or you may think of a *treatment regimen you're supposed to be following,* but lately have become lax or stopped completely (eg, erratic diet or exercise program, medication you're not taking regularly, strengthening/stretching exercises you've been skipping, etc).

➤ Now, write down your health concern, along with a few notes about its underlying threat to your health. What is your self-care history with this problem. What might be the consequences if you don't take action? Are you worried about some specific disease? Or the length or quality of your life? What have you done about the problem in the past?

   ☞ *For each of the next four steps, allow people plenty of time to consider their ranking before you make the corresponding explanatory comment. Add some examples of your own to bring the categories alive.*

➤ Now rate your judgment of the *severity* of this health concern on a 1 to 5 scale where:

1 = very minor;
5 = a life and death issue.

Severity can be determined by the amount of pain, its duration, the degree of disability it causes you or the impact it has on your activities, lifestyle and friendships. Write down the word *severity* and your ranking.

● **Generally, the less severe we judge the problem to be, the less likely we are to do something about it.** The more severe we believe the problem is, the more likely we will be to take action—unless it's a #5 life and death issue, which we might ignore because we are afraid of what we might find out.

➤ Next, rate your judgment of how *susceptible* you are to this problem or the consequences of not taking action (eg, if you don't start exercising, how susceptible might you be to gaining weight, depression, cardiovascular disease, etc). Again, use a 1 to 5 scale. Write down the word *susceptible* and your ranking:

1 = it's very unlikely I would have this problem;
5 = it's almost certain I have or will develop this problem.

● **Susceptibility is a** *subjective* **belief about how likely you are to have or to develop the problem.** Usually the more susceptible you believe you are, the more likely you are to try to take care of the problem. Even in the face of mounting evidence to the contrary, most of us do little about a potential health problem if we believe we are not susceptible.

➤ Next, list the *barriers* that keep you from taking the recommended health action for your concern. Then rate the *impact of these barriers* using a 1 to 5 scale:

1 = the barriers hinder my action very little;
5 = the barriers make it almost impossible for me to act.

● Typical barriers include perceptions such as "It costs too much," "It takes too long," "No one else around me does it," "I don't like doing it," etc. **The fewer or less potent the perceived barriers, the more likely it is that we will take appropriate action.** As the perceived power of the barriers goes up, the likelihood of action decreases.

➤ Now rate on a 1 to 5 scale the *benefits* you believe you would experience if you did take appropriate health-related actions.

> *1 = I don't think it will help a bit;*
>
> *5 = I know it will have a dramatic, immediate, positive effect.*

- **When we believe the action won't make much difference, we're not likely to do anything.** The likelihood of our following through on self-care plans increases when we believe more positively about their potential benefits to us.

4) The trainer invites the group to reflect on their responses to the major issues of this health belief model.

✔ Given your view of 1) the **Severity of your problem**, 2) how **Susceptible you believe you are**, 3) the **Barriers that stop you**, and 4) the **Benefits you expect**—is it any wonder that you have not yet taken any effective action to respond to this problem or to solve it?

5) The trainer challenges participants to review each of their rankings and write down some alternative beliefs they could cultivate in each area to promote more responsible self-care.

☞ *Allow 2–3 minutes for this reflection. If necessary, prompt the group with a few thought-provoking questions (eg, How severe is the problem, really? How susceptible are you? Would your family or physician agree? Can you overcome and minimize some of the barriers that keep you from acting? Can you improve your outlook on the benefits you would expect to receive by this action?).*

6) The trainer solicits examples of health concerns chosen by participants and their old and new beliefs. She uses these contributions to illustrate and reinforce a closing peptalk.

- **Information is not enough.** Good intentions and will power are not enough. Beliefs and actions are what really count if we want to maximize our health and vitality.

- **When you want to *help encourage yourself to act*,** don't just grit your teeth and try will power alone. Rather give yourself a boost by altering the four health beliefs. Then your follow through will become much easier.

VARIATIONS

■ Following *Step 3*, the group could brainstorm ways of improving the likelihood of their positive follow through; or participants could share their observations with each other in small groups.

Planning
& Closure

130 BEAT THE ODDS

In this simple closing, participants remember key ideas, reflect on self-care strengths and weaknesses, and identify new behaviors and attitudes they plan to implement.

GOALS

To reinforce key concepts and increase transfer of learning.

To affirm self-care strengths and pinpoint areas for growth and change.

GROUP SIZE

Unlimited.

TIME FRAME

10–15 minutes

MATERIALS NEEDED

Beat the Odds worksheets and blank 3x5 index cards for everyone.

PROCESS

1) The trainer begins by announcing statistics about the long term impact of learning experiences like this one:
   - If this is an average group, by tomorrow people in this room will remember about 75% of what they have heard here.
   - By the next day 50% of the content will be forgotten, and 85% will be lost within 4 days.
   - In two weeks, the average person will remember only 2% of what was heard today.

2) The trainer notes that these statistics can be improved immensely if people actively use the information right away and continue to review and apply their learnings.

   She challenges the group to beat the odds by using the information and skills they have learned as soon as possible (eg, sharing an insight, trying a new skill, making a desired change, affirming a new awareness, etc).

3) The trainer distributes **Beat the Odds** worksheets and 3x5 cards to all. Participants record their strengths and weaknesses, plans for change, and key ideas. (5 minutes)

4) Participants take turns sharing from their 3x5 cards key ideas they want to remember. After everyone has taken a turn, the trainer encourages participants to put the card where they will see it several times a day to reinforce what they have learned and extend the impact of the workshop experience.

TRAINER'S NOTES

Submitted by Pat Miller.

BEAT THE ODDS

One value of a workshop is to remind you of your strengths—*what you are already doing right*. You will want to continue these behaviors and develop them further. What self-care strengths do you want to affirm and continue?

STRENGTHS

In light of what you have learned here, are there any self-care weaknesses that deserve your attention? What new attitudes or behaviors will diminish those weaknesses?

WEAKNESS   NEW ATTITUDE OR BEHAVIOR

On the 3x5 card provided, write down the key ideas you want to remember from this workshop.

131 DISCOVERIES

Throughout the learning experience and between sessions, participants capture their insights in a journal and periodically translate these discoveries into concrete goals.

GOALS

To keep track of key ideas and personal discoveries during the learning experience.

To apply insights to life situations and develop a plan for implementing healthy changes.

GROUP SIZE

Unlimited.

TIME FRAME

5 minutes at the beginning of the session; 1–2 minutes at several points in the session; 10–15 minutes at closing.

MATERIALS NEEDED

Journal or notebook for each participant; One or more copies of the **Discoveries** worksheet for each person.

PROCESS

1) Before the session begins, the trainer distributes a journal to each participant and explains the guidelines for its use:
   - The purpose of this journal is to record your discoveries and insights about wellness throughout today's session(s). At various points during the session, we'll take a couple of minutes to write down our discoveries. These discoveries are a personal record of what you're learning about your own wellness. You may have several insights each time we pause.
   - Some discoveries may be minor bits of information like the number of calories burned per mile of walking or the salt content of a can of soup. Other discoveries may be of major importance such as your personal health risk status, or the impact of stress on your blood pressure, or the assessment that you may be dependent on alcohol,

or the discovery that other people have had feelings and experiences similar to your own.

➤ At the top of the first page, write: *"I am discovering that . . ."* Use this phrase to stimulate your thinking whenever we stop to record our insights and discoveries.

➤ Write the number "1" directly beneath the heading. Now you have prepared a space for your first discovery. Each insight you write down should be numbered. When you have finished recording one discovery, write the number for the next one. The idea is to encourage yourself to always be on the alert for another insight.

2) Periodically throughout the session(s) (eg, after a content presentation, worksheet reflection, or small group discussion), the trainer asks participants to record in their journals what they are discovering about their own wellness as a result of the process.

☞ *Allow 1–2 minutes at each checkpoint for recording discoveries.*

3) At the end of the session, the trainer asks the participants to look over their journals and decide which discoveries deserve further attention.

➤ Review all the discoveries in your journal. As you read, circle any significant, surprising or important items (eg, "my salt intake is way too high" or "breast cancer is the greatest health risk factor in my age bracket").

➤ Then look back over the items you highlighted and transfer the most important discoveries from your journal onto the left column of the worksheet, marked *Discovery,* one insight per box. Try to narrow down your choices; undertaking too many changes at once can be difficult and self-defeating.

☞ *Allow enough time for participants to review their notes and transfer the discoveries. If you have time, distribute several worksheets to each person so they can transfer more than three discoveries.*

If people start to get restless, move on to the next step. Encourage those who are not yet finished to stop and apply the next step to one of their discoveries so they understand the process. They can then finish reviewing their journals later.

4) The trainer makes the following points about lifestyle changes, asking participants to consider how these principles might apply to the discoveries they have written on their worksheets:

- Building a healthier lifestyle involves reducing or eliminating negative behaviors—and increasing or adding positive behaviors.
- Daily routines and choices have a cumulative impact on wellness. "Drastic" changes are often the long-term result of small daily choices. One doughnut won't kill anyone—but a doughnut every day for years can pose a health hazard. An occasional walk around the block won't add much to your fitness level, but a 30-minute walk every day could add years to your life.

5) The trainer instructs participants to reflect on the *first discovery on their list* and consider how they can turn this insight into positive behavior that will increase their well-being.

> ➤ In the middle column, jot a few notes about what this insight means in your life by finishing the sentence: *"I need to . . ."*
>
> The purpose of this step is to translate the insight into a goal. At this point, the goal may be somewhat vague (eg, "I need to cut down on my salt intake," or "I need to take precautions about breast cancer").

6) As soon as most people have identified some "need-to's" the trainer challenges participants to formulate concrete goals.

> ➤ Refine each *"I need to . . ."* statement into a series of specific behavioral steps you can take to apply this discovery to your life and lifestyle (eg, "I will use salt substitute in cooking, leave the salt shaker off the table and snack on pretzels instead of chips," or "I will schedule a mammogram, swallow my embarrassment and ask for specific instructions on breast self-examinations, and check out my family history").
>
> ➤ Write the steps of your plan in the third column, marked *"I will . . ."*

7) *Steps 5* and *6* are repeated for the other discoveries on the worksheet.

> ☞ *If time is short, suggest that participants finish the worksheet by themselves after the session.*

8) In closing, the trainer asks group members to volunteer examples from their worksheets. Participants read their discovery, their "I need to . . ." statement, and their "I will . . ." steps.

VARIATIONS

■ As part of *Step 8*, participants could gather in small groups to compare discoveries and share their resolutions for change.

TRAINER'S NOTES

DISCOVERIES

DISCOVERY	I NEED TO . . .	I WILL . . .

DISCOVERIES

DISCOVERY	I NEED TO . . .	I WILL . . .

132 GIFTS

In this closing ritual participants "take the wraps off" and affirm the benefits gained from their study together.

GOALS

To provide group closure.

To reinforce learnings and affirm insights.

To give feedback to the trainer.

GROUP SIZE

Unlimited.

TIME FRAME

5–15 minutes

MATERIALS NEEDED

One gift box for each group of 4 participants.

> ☞ *Prepare the gift boxes in advance with at least 5 layers of colorful wrapping paper (or if you plan larger groups, one more layer than the number of people in the group). To spice up the action, use boxes of different sizes and a wide variety of seasonal and special occasion gift wraps. Make sure the outside layer is different on each gift.*

PROCESS

1) The trainer instructs participants to rejoin their small groups (or form new 4-person groups) for a special closing ritual.

2) After everyone is settled, the trainer distributes a gift box to each group and gives instructions for unwrapping.

   ➤ The person holding the present now begins by carefully taking the outside layer of paper off.

   ➤ As you are unwrapping, describe to the other people in your group one gift you've received in this learning experience (eg, an insight, a new perspective, information, motivation, new friendship, etc). Describe the gift in detail—and with enthusiasm and energetic exclamations of appreciation.

> When you're finished, give the present to someone else to unwrap and describe a gift they have received here.

> Each person should take about one minute to unwrap and describe your gift of learning. I'll interrupt and let you know when the time is half up.

3) The trainer gives a warning at the halfway point and after the groups have finished their gift sharing, he gives directions for the final step.

> Now it's time to give a gift in return.

> Take two minutes together in your group to decide on a symbolic gift of appreciation you would like to give to someone in the room, or to the entire group. Once your have chosen a recipient and composed an appropriate affirmation, pick a spokesperson to make your presentation.

4) The trainer calls on the groups one by one. The spokesperson gives the gift and affirms why it is deserved by the recipient(s).

☞ *Be prepared to graciously accept a few of these yourself. Enjoy the fruits of your labor—you deserve it!*

VARIATION

■ In a particularly cohesive group, when there are 15 or fewer participants, use only one gift (wrapped with the appropriate number of layers). This process will take longer (about 20 minutes), but allows an opportunity for everyone to have a final good-bye contact with each other.

TRAINER'S NOTES

This process is adapted from an exercise described in Group Magazine.

©1994 Whole Person Press 210 W Michigan Duluth MN 55802   (800) 247-6789

133 A WORK OF ART

In this closing summary, participants create personal "pop art" sculptures symbolizing their enlightened understanding of wellness.

GOALS

To articulate insights gained and to provide closure to the learning experience.

To provide a visual and tactile form for participants to express wellness as they now understand it.

GROUP SIZE

Unlimited.

TIME FRAME

30 minutes

MATERIALS NEEDED

Various arts and crafts supplies, including any or all of the following: paper plates, paper clips, paper or foam cups, cotton balls, straws, colored felt, string/yarn, balloons, construction paper, ribbons, tissue paper, tongue depressors, felt-tipped markers or crayons, pipe cleaners, sequins or glitter, scissors, adhesive tape, glue or paste, newsprint.

PROCESS

☞ *For this exercise, you can use groups that were assembled for other exercises. Members will complete their sculptures alone, then share them with the group.*

1) The trainer distributes materials to each of the groups.

☞ *It is not necessary to distribute identical materials to each group. If one group complains that another group got better materials, remind them that we are all born with advantages and disadvantages. Wellness is what we make of the materials we've been given.*

2) The trainer tells participants that they will each make a sculpture representing their conceptualization of wellness, using the following guidelines:

➤ Take a couple of minutes to think about what it means to be well. Think about it not in words, but in colors, shapes and textures. Is it soft and fluffy, smooth and shiny? Is it red or green or a combination of colors? Has your conceptualization of wellness changed, based on what you've learned today in this course/session/workshop?

➤ Wellness is an entirely original creation; it's not the same for any two people. Use the materials provided to make a sculpture that represents your concept of wellness.

☞ *If participants say things like, "I'm not an artist," tell them, "Just think of all the times you've seen a piece of modern sculpture and said, 'I can do better than that!'" Remind them that what's important is not how it looks, but what it means to them.*

Allow 10 minutes or so for people to create sculptures. If people say they're not finished when the time is up, remind them that wellness is an ongoing project.

3) The trainer instructs participants to describe their sculptures to the group. Explain the choice of materials and colors, and what the sculpture means to them.

VARIATIONS

■ If there are fewer than fifteen participants, do not divide them into smaller groups. In *Step 3*, participants describe their sculptures to the entire group.

■ Instead of offering a variety of supplies, give each participant a limited supply of one of the following materials to make their sculpture:

Clay or Play-Doh. One long stick of clay or half a can of Play-Doh (enough to make a ball the size of a small tangerine).

Pipe cleaners, one pack per participant.

First-aid supplies. A dozen tongue depressors, a role of adhesive tape or assorted Band-Aids.

Potato or soap. Distribute a small paring knife or pen knife to each person, along with a potato or bar of soap to carve. Caution: This one can be messy! Provide paper towels and cleanup materials.

©1994 Whole Person Press 210 W Michigan Duluth MN 55802   (800) 247-6789

TRAINER'S NOTES

134 WHISPER CIRCLE

In this affirming small-group activity, participants are quietly showered with positive feedback.

GOALS

To promote group cohesiveness and provide closure.

To allow and encourage group members to provide positive feedback for each other.

GROUP SIZE

Unlimited.

TIME FRAME

10–15 minutes

PROCESS

1) The trainer asks participants to rejoin their small groups for a closing ceremony.

   ☞ *This process works best with participants who have interacted and shared significantly with each other. Groups need to have at least six people to maximize the variety of feedback, so combine two or three groups if necessary to create groups of 6–12 persons each.*

2) As soon as everyone is settled, the trainer gives instructions for the *Whisper Circle.*

   ➤ Stand close together, facing each other in a circle. You will take turns standing in the middle of your group to receive positive feedback from the others.

   ➤ Group members in the circle will *whisper affirmations* to the member standing in the middle. Everyone should participate in showering the center person with compliments.

   It is not necessary to take turns—just try to keep the whispers flowing one right after another. The idea is to surround the person in the middle with a continuous stream of positive feedback for two minutes. If you run out of ideas, repeat your favorites.

➤ Be sure that your affirmations are positive, personal and sincere. Sarcasm and humor are inappropriate. If possible, the affirmations should reflect something you have observed about this person today.

☞ *Give some specific examples (eg, "Your smile sure lights up your face," or "I've noticed how carefully you listen to others," or "You've made some courageous decisions," etc).*

➤ When you are the person in the middle, keep your eyes closed and listen attentively to all the positive strokes you will receive. Just soak up all those affirmations—and enjoy it.

➤ Decide now who will be first and then start your whispering. Keep it up non-stop until I interrupt and tell you to switch to the next person.

3) Every 2 minutes the trainer stops the process and invites a different group member to step into the middle of the *Whisper Circle*. This step is repeated until all have taken a turn.

4) In closing, the trainer reconvenes the entire group and poses one or more of the following questions for discussion.

✔ How did it feel to be the person in the middle?

✔ Is it easier to accept affirmations when they are given anonymously? Is it easier to offer them anonymously?

✔ Did this technique bring out affirmations that you might not otherwise have given?

✔ What were some of the benefits of today's session?

Submitted by Sondra Smalley.

©1994 Whole Person Press 210 W Michigan Duluth MN 55802   (800) 247-6789

Group
Energizers

135 12 DAYS OF WELLNESS

Participants join in a carol celebrating the joys of wellness.

GOALS

To reinforce wellness concepts.

To provide an energy break.

GROUP SIZE

Unlimited.

TIME FRAME

5 minutes

MATERIALS NEEDED

Newsprint poster, overhead transparency or handout with the **12 Days of Wellness** lyrics.

PROCESS

1) The trainer invites participants to join in a hymn to wellness, using new words to a familiar Christmas carol.

   ☞ *With a large group, divide into 11 groups of roughly the same number of people. Assign each group a number from 2 to 12. Everyone sings the first verse together (and subsequent occurrences of the line "and a hammock in a shade tree"). Other lines are sung each time by the group with the corresponding number.*

VARIATIONS

■ The lyrics may be adapted/edited to fit your audience. Or let the group rewrite the lyrics to match your course content or setting.

Submitted by Juile Lusk. This ditty was one of the theme songs for Roanoke Valley: Alive and Well Week 1987.

THE 12 DAYS OF WELLNESS

On the FIRST day of wellness, my true love gave to me . . .
A HAMMOCK IN A SHADE TREE.

On the SECOND day of wellness, my true love gave to me . . .
TWO AEROBIC SHOES . . .
and a hammock in a shade tree.

On the THIRD day of wellness, my true love gave to me . . .
THREE SQUARE MEALS . . .
two aerobic shoes and a hammock in a shade tree.

On the FOURTH day of wellness, my true love gave to me . . .
FOUR FOOD GROUPS . . .
three square meals, two aerobic shoes
and a hammock in a shade tree.

On the FIFTH day of wellness, my true love gave to me . . .
FIVE HUGS—NOT DRUGS . . .
four food groups, three square meals, two aerobic shoes
and a hammock in a shade tree.

On the SIXTH day of wellness, my true love gave to me . . .
SIX VEGGIES STEAMING . . .

On the SEVENTH day of wellness, my true love gave to me . . .
SEVEN DAYS FOR PRAYING . . .

On the EIGHTH day of wellness, my true love gave to me . . .
EIGHT HOURS FOR SLEEPING . . .

On the NINTH day of wellness, my true love gave to me . . .
NINE LAUGHS FROM JOKING . . .

On the TENTH day of wellness my true love gave to me . . .
TEN TOES FOR WALKING . . .

On the ELEVENTH day of wellness my true love gave to me . . .
ELEVEN DAYS—NO SMOKING . . .

On the TWELFTH day of wellness my true love gave to me . . .
TWELVE FRIENDS FOR TALKING . . .
Eleven days—no smoking . . .
Ten toes for walking . . .
Nine laughs from joking . . .
Eight hours for sleeping . . .
Seven days for praying . . .
Six veggies steaming . . .
Five hugs—not drugs . . .
Four food groups . . .
Three square meals . . .
Two aerobic shoes . . .
And a hammock in a shade tree.

Original lyrics by Dr Dan Davidson.

©1994 Whole Person Press 210 W Michigan Duluth MN 55802   (800) 247-6789

136 ALL EARS

Participants use different types of ear massage to energize themselves.

GOALS

To learn a simple self-care technique for stimulating body systems.

GROUP SIZE

Unlimited.

TIME FRAME

5 minutes

PROCESS

1) The trainer invites participants to join in a self-care routine that the Chinese have used for 5,000 years to get their energies moving again. He then guides them through one or more of the ear massages described below:

   ➤ Make a "V" with your first two fingers and slide your hand up along the side of your head until your ear is surrounded by the "V" of your fingers. Vigorously massage all the area around the ear.

   ➤ Now massage your ears themselves with thumb and forefinger. Roll the outer edge between your fingers. Stretch it, pull it gently, pinch and rub it. Then massage the inner ridge. And finally the inner area.

   ➤ Use your whole hand to rub the ear forward and backward vigorously several times.

   ➤ To stimulate hearing, cover one ear with the opposite palm and tap lightly on the back of the hand with your fingers. Repeat with the other ear.

Submitted by Larry Tobin.

137 AS THE SEASONS TURN

In this series of gentle yoga stretches, participants use images of nature to help them relax.

GOALS

To release tension through conscious breathing and movement.

To promote relaxation and centering through balancing and imagery.

GROUP SIZE

Unlimited.

TIME FRAME

5 minutes

PROCESS

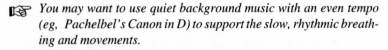 *You may want to use quiet background music with an even tempo (eg, Pachelbel's Canon in D) to support the slow, rhythmic breathing and movements.*

1) The leader demonstrates the **As the Seasons Turn** stretch movements and guides participants through the cycle of the seasons several times.

Submitted by Martha Belknap.

AS THE SEASONS TURN Script

SPRING

Stand with knees relaxed and your hands resting in front of your pelvis.

Imagine a strong oak tree with its roots reaching deep into the earth in **springtime.**

Inhale as you draw up nutrients from the soil—up through the trunk of the tree, out to reach all the branches rising toward the sun as you **raise your arms** overhead.

SUMMER

With your **arms stretched overhead,**

Imagine the tree at its peak of fullness in the middle of **summer.**

Exhale as you extend the branches to the side **stretching your arms wide** to the side at shoulder height.

Inhale as you reach the branches upward again **raising your arms.**

AUTUMN

Make your tree very tall, with your **thumbs linked overhead,**

Imagine the west winds of **autumn.**

Exhale as the tree **bends** to one side.

Inhale and lift to center.

Exhale as the tree **bends** to the other side.

Inhale and lift to center.

Exhale as the leaves are blown to the ground and you **drop your hands** to your sides.

WINTER

With your **hands clasped** behind your seat,

Imagine the branches of the tree laden with fresh snow in **winter.**

Inhale as you **lift your arms** behind you.

Exhale as the tree bends forward, lowering its branches toward the ground.

Inhale and lift to the center position, then **relax your arms.**

138 CLAPDANCE

This peppy movement routine incorporates rhythm, cooperation and interaction.

GOALS

To loosen up the group and get people together.

To provide an opportunity for playful interaction.

GROUP SIZE

Works best with 25 or more people.

TIME FRAME

5–10 minutes

MATERIALS NEEDED

Large room with movable chairs or plenty of open space to "dance;" tape recorder and lively music with a regular beat (folk music, square dance tunes or marches); **Seated** and **Circle Clapdance** instructions.

PROCESS

☞ *Be sure to practice the **Clapdance** sequences several times by yourself and with a group of guinea pigs so that you can demonstrate without notes—and with great enthusiasm. Your role here is like that of a square dance caller, so ham it up and play the part. Using a microphone and a sing-song voice adds to the folk dance atmosphere.*

1) At a point in the session when people have been sitting for a long period without interaction, the trainer turns on the music and leads participants through the Seated Clapdance routine.

   ☞ *It's best to just get the group started without much introduction. The process itself is contagious, but with a more formal audience you may have to repeat the first few sequences a couple of times and chide people to get with it (eg, "This is a required playtime for all workaholics").*

2) At the end of the *Seated Clapdance*, the trainer invites people to stand and keep clapping in unison as they join him in the open space and make a circle.

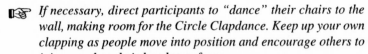

> ☞ *If necessary, direct participants to "dance" their chairs to the wall, making room for the Circle Clapdance. Keep up your own clapping as people move into position and encourage others to join you when their hands are free.*

3) As soon as all participants are gathered in a circle, the trainer guides the group through the Circle Clapdance sequence.

VARIATIONS

■ If no music is available, try this exercise *a capella*. Use a familiar tune with an 8-beat count (eg, *Row Row Row Your Boat, Frere Jacques*, etc). Sing the song together and clap with the beat.

SEATED CLAPDANCE Instructions

Raise your right hand; Raise your left hand.
Put your hands together (clap above head).
Now clap high four times.

Now clap your thighs twice;
And clap in front twice (chest high);
Clap high twice;
And clap your thighs twice.

Now clap with one hand to each of your neighbors twice;
And clap high twice;
Then clap hands twice with your neighbors again;
And clap your thighs twice.

> ☞ *Keep up your clapping rhythm as you tell people that for the next step they will need to get some legs next to them! Encourage people to move close enough to reach their neighbors' thighs.*

Everyone ready? Clap your own thighs twice;
Now clap the thigh of the person to your left with your left hand while you clap your own left thigh with your right hand;
Clap your own thighs twice again;
Then clap the thigh of your right-hand neighbor with your right hand while you clap your own right thigh with your left hand.

> ☞ *For best effect, repeat this sequence again saying something like, "Okay, this time for keeps—anyone who goofs up will have to go stand in the corner!"*

©1994 Whole Person Press 210 W Michigan Duluth MN 55802   (800) 247-6789

Now a final round:
Clap up twice;
Clap hands with your neighbors twice;
Cross your hands and clap both your neighbors' thighs;
Clap your own thighs twice.

Now, stand up and clap front eight times;
And give yourselves an ovation!

CIRCLE CLAPDANCE Instructions

Let's join hands and circle right (8 counts)
Then circle left (8 counts)

Now everyone in to the center and raise your hands (4 counts)
and back out again (4 counts);
Now in again with arms up and a great big WHOOP! (4 counts)
and back out again (4 counts).

> ☞ *Repeat this sequence two or three times, then ask partici-*
> *pants to pair up with a neighbor and promenade in the*
> *circle for 8 counts.*

Now face your partner for the claps.
Clap high twice;
Clap in front twice;
Clap your thighs twice;
And clap front twice again.

Let's try that again.

> ☞ *Repeat the sequence twice, then ask the pairs to pair up in*
> *quartets and make squares, with partners facing each*
> *other.*

Now this will take some coordination:
One pair should start down, clapping their thighs, while the other pair starts
up, clapping high.

Clap high twice (one pair), low twice (other pair);
Clap front twice (both pairs);
Clap low twice (one pair), high twice (other pair);
Clap front twice (both pairs).

> ☞ *Repeat this clapping several times and close with a final*
> *circle dance with loud WHOOPS!*

Submitted by Glenn Q Bannerman.

---

139 FIT AS A FIDDLE

This light-hearted poem pokes fun at the self-righteousness of the wellness movement.

GOALS

To put wellness in perspective.

GROUP SIZE

Unlimited.

TIME FRAME

5 minutes

PROCESS

1) The trainer chooses an appropriate moment (eg, just before a break, at the end of a serious content segment, before a presentation on the importance of compassion as a component of wellness, etc) and reads the **Fit as a Fiddle** poem to the group.

FIT AS A FIDDLE Script

They brush and they floss with care every day,
But not before breakfast of both curds and whey.

He jogs for his heart, she bikes for her nerves;
They assert themselves daily with appropriate verve.

He is loving and tender and caring and kind,
Not one chauvinist thought is allowed in his mind.

They are slim and attractive, well-dressed and just fun.
They are strong and well-immunized against everything under the sun.

They are sparkling and lively and having a ball.
Their diet's high fiber and low cholesterol.

Cocktails are avoided in favor of juice;
Cigarettes are shunned as one would the noose.

They drive their car safely with belts well in place;
At home not one hazard ever will they face.

1.2 children they raise, both sharing the job.
One is named Betty, point two is named Bob.

And when, at the age of two hundred and three,
they jog from this life to one still MORE free,

They'll pass through those portals to claim their reward
and St Peter will stop them, "JUST FOR A WORD."

"What HO!" he will say, "You cannot go in.
This place is reserved for those without sin."

"But we've followed the rules," she'll say with a fright,
"We're healthy—near perfect—and incredibly bright."

"But that's it," will say Peter, drawing himself tall,
"You've missed the point of living by thinking so small.

"Life is more than health habits, though useful they be;
It is purpose and meaning, the grand mystery.

"You've discovered a part of what makes humans whole,
and mistaken that part for the shape of the soul.

"You are fitter than fiddles and sound as a bell,
Self-righteous, intolerant and boring as hell!"

By William H Carlyon, Director, Department of Health Education, American Medical Association.

140 JOKE AROUND

Participants join in a hilarious interpersonal contact sport.

GOALS

To demonstrate the power of humor as a healthy mood-altering activity.

To promote group interaction.

GROUP SIZE

Unlimited.

TIME FRAME

5 minutes

PROCESS

1) The trainer introduces the exercise with a few comments on the power and value of humor in healthy relationships.

   - **Humor is a natural tension reliever.** Tense situations can often be defused with a delightful joke. Humor often provides a fresh perspective that frees people to change their expectations or give up entrenched positions. Especially in intimate relationships, humor can help us through tense moments.

   - **Humor brings people together.** Laughter is a universal form of communication that is contagious and easy to share. Victor Borge captured the essence of humor in this aphorism: "Laughter is the shortest distance between two people."

2) The trainer asks participants to recall a favorite joke, cartoon or amusing anecdote.

   ☞ *Tell a few jokes of your own to stimulate the group, or use these two:*

     + *There was a news report last week about a small town that experienced an extraordinary robbery. "It was reported to-day that vandals made off with all the toilet seats at the local police station. The police have nothing to go on."*

     + *Did you hear the one about the magician who walked down the street and turned into a drugstore?*

Then encourage participants to remember knock-knock jokes, puns, cartoons, malapropisms, witty bumper stickers, funny stories from children—anything humorous. Caution against long, shaggy-dog stories and any kind of put-down humor (eg, ethnic, racist, sexist, etc).

3) After a moment for reflection, participants are instructed to stand and find a partner—preferably someone they don't know well. Pairs tell each other a favorite joke.

4) The trainer announces that telling jokes is more fun with a larger audience. He instructs each pair to find two other pairs and form groups of six.

As soon as groups are settled, the trainer gives instructions for the second round.

➤ Go around the group and take turns telling your jokes or amusing stories. You can tell the same joke you just told your partner (maybe this time you'll get the punch line straight!) Or feel free to tell a different one. Remember, you don't have to be Johnny Carson, just do you best to deliver your joke with enthusiasm and humor.

☞ *You may want to have some jokes or cartoons available for participants who panic.*

➤ When someone else is telling a joke, the rest of the group should allow yourselves to be tickled. Let the humor touch you. Laugh if possible. No moans, groans, sarcasm or disparaging remarks.

5) As the laughter begins to die down, the trainer reconvenes the group and asks for a few examples of the very best jokes.

Submitted by Joel Goodman.

©1994 Whole Person Press 210 W Michigan Duluth MN 55802   (800) 247-6789

141 NEW SICK LEAVE POLICY

This humorous reading spoofs the "blame the victim" attitude taken by some sick leave policies.

GOALS

To provide an amusing look at a serious subject.

GROUP SIZE

Unlimited.

TIME FRAME

5 minutes

MATERIALS NEEDED

New Sick Leave Policy script.

PROCESS

1) The trainer introduces the policy with a tongue-in-cheek "announcement" tailored to fit the audience (eg, "Since we've got everyone together in one room, management has asked me to read an important memo").

2) The trainer reads the **New Sick Leave Policy** script.

Joel Goodman brought this anonymous piece to our attention. If anyone knows the original source, please let us know.

©1994 Whole Person Press 210 W Michigan Duluth MN 55802   (800) 247-6789

NEW SICK LEAVE POLICY

The management wholeheartedly endorses the wellness movement, particularly the idea that we can all take responsibility for our own health. To reflect this enlightened attitude, the company has instituted a new sick leave policy for employees, as follows:

SICKNESS:

There is no excuse. We will no longer accept a doctor's statement as proof, as we believe that if you are able to go to the doctor, you are able to come to work. What's more, if you took care of yourself in the first place, you wouldn't be sick.

LEAVE OF ABSENCE FOR AN OPERATION:

We are no longer allowing this practice. We wish to discourage any thought that you may have about needing an operation. We believe that as long as you are employed here, you will need all of whatever parts you have and should not consider having any of them removed. We hired you as you are and to have anything removed would certainly make you less than we bargained for.

RESTROOM BREAKS:

Too much time is being spent in the restroom. In the future, we will follow the practice of going to the restroom in alphabetical order. For instance, those whose names begin with "A" will go from 8 a.m. to 8:15 a.m., "B" will go from 8:15 to 8:30 a.m., and so on. If you are unable to go at your time, you will have to wait until the day when your turn comes again.

DEATH (OTHER THAN YOUR OWN):

This is no excuse. There is nothing you can do for them, and we are sure that someone else in a lesser position can attend to the arrangements. However, if the funeral can be held in late afternoon, we will be glad to let you off one hour early, provided that your share of work is ahead enough to keep the job going in your absence.

DEATH (YOUR OWN):

This will be accepted as an excuse, but we would like a two-week notice, as we feel it is your duty to teach someone else your job.

142 ON PURPOSE

Participants discover the power of purpose during this exercise in concentration and repetition.

GOALS

To explore the role of intentionality in healthy lifestyle choices.

GROUP SIZE

Unlimited.

TIME FRAME

10 minutes

MATERIALS NEEDED

Large clock with a sweep secondhand.

PROCESS

1) The trainer begins with a few comments on the role of "purpose" in our lives.

   - **Purpose is at the very center of our lives**—of our lifestyle choices. Doing something "on purpose" suggests that we are making a *choice* and are *moving toward* something we desire or believe in.
   - Acting "on purpose" is a joyful undertaking when we are aware of where we are headed and why.
   - **We can train our will power and concentration** so that we can be "on purpose" in more areas of life—especially those choices that lead to longer, healthier lives.

2) The trainer invites participants to join in a series of experiments that illustrate the power of purpose. She guides the group through the three exercises outlined below.

   ➤ First, start tapping your pen or pencil on a hard surface (table, book, chair).
   ➤ For the next two minutes concentrate on the tip of your pen hitting the surface each time and try to keep in rhythm with me and the rest of the group.

☞ *Once the group is going, do not distract them with any more verbal instructions. Just concentrate on keeping your tapping rhythm even and regular. After 2 minutes announce the next activity.*

➤ Now we will try another intentional exercise. This time we will purposefully get up from our chairs and then sit down again—in rhythm—for two minutes.

➤ Concentrate on the process of standing up and sitting down. Be on purpose and focus on what you're doing. If your mind wanders, refocus on the rhythm of getting up and down.

☞ *Set a slow, rhythmic pace as you stand and sit. Keep time and introduce the next step after 2 minutes.*

➤ This time we will focus our attention on time. Watch the second hand on the clock go around for two minutes.

➤ Concentrate on the tip of the second hand and try to stay *on purpose.* If extraneous thoughts arise, just let them go and refocus your attention on the purpose of this exercise—to follow the second hand as it sweeps around two full revolutions. (2 minutes)

3) After the third exercise is finished, the trainer solicits observations from the group on the nature and experience of purpose.

4) In closing, the trainer invites participants to focus on a particular health-related behavior they would like to target for *on purpose* action in the day or weeks ahead (eg, breathing, eating, forgiveness, exercise, gratitude, etc).

● Concentrating on a meaningless task demonstrates the potential power of purposeful choices in more meaningful areas of life.

● We can *practice* being *on purpose.* As we build up our ability to concentrate, we increase our commitment to our choices and enhance the likelihood that we can make significant behavior and lifestyle changes.

Submitted by Neil Young.

143 SENSORY RELAXATION

Participants focus on sensory awareness in this suggestive relaxation routine.

GOALS

To reduce tension through the use of imagination and attention to sensation.

TIME FRAME

5-10 minutes

MATERIALS NEEDED

Sensory Relaxation Suggestions.

☞ *You may want to provide some relaxing New Age music as a background for this experience (eg, Steve Halpern, Georgia Kelly, Kitaro, Windham Hill artists, etc).*

PROCESS

1) The trainer invites participants to prepare for an unusual relaxation experience.

➤ Find a comfortable position.

➤ I will be reading a number of suggestions that will require that you use your imagination to tune in to your sensations.

➤ There is no right or wrong way to respond. Just listen to each statement and allow yourself to respond naturally. Don't try to make anything happen. Simply notice your sensations.

☞ *You may need to caution participants not to respond verbally. This is an exercise in imagination!*

2) The trainer reads some or all of the **Sensory Relaxation Suggestions**, pausing 15 seconds between each statement so participants can attend to the suggested sensation.

☞ *In your sequence be sure to include the first two and the last four suggestions.*

3) The trainer solicits a few reactions to the process from the group.

SENSORY RELAXATION SUGGESTIONS Script

☞ *pause 15 seconds after each statement*

Gently let your eyes close. (pause)

Allow yourself to sit heavily in your chair. (pause)

Can you imagine the space between your ears?

Become aware of the distance between your ears.

Can you become aware of how close your breath comes to the back of your eyes every time you inhale?

Become aware of the space within your mouth.

Notice the position of your tongue within your mouth.

Can you feel your lips becoming soft?

Can you imagine a warm spring breeze against your cheek?

Can you imagine the sun radiating on the back of your neck?

Can you expand that warmth down your entire back?

Can you feel the weight of your arms pulling down your shoulders?

Can you become aware of one of your arms being more relaxed than the other?

Can you feel the space between your fingers?

Can you feel a warm breeze brush against your fingers?

Can you make your legs feel as limp as a rag doll?

Can you feel the floor beneath your feet?

Try to feel like you are becoming a few inches taller by allowing yourself to stretch out through the bottom of your feet.

Can you imagine that your arms are growing?

As you inhale, pretend that the air is puffing you up like a balloon; as you exhale, feel like a balloon that is slowly losing its air.

Now picture your lungs as birds wings.
As you slowly inhale, picture the wings rising gracefully.
As you slowly exhale, imagine the wings lowering smoothly.

Can you feel yourself floating as if on a cloud?

Can you imagine that you are looking at something that is very far away?

Can you imagine in your mind's eye a beautiful object suspended a few feet in front of you?

Can you imagine that you can hear a seashell at your ear?

Try to imagine your head sinking into a soft, fluffy pillow.
Check to see if your feel tension anywhere in your body.
Send mental messages to those areas to eliminate the tension.
As you inhale, imagine your breath is sending energy to all areas of your body.
As you exhale, imagine any tension is leaving your body through your fingertips and toes.

Can you allow yourself to sit where you are and enjoy your state of relaxation? (longer pause)

Can you allow your eyes to open? Open them now, and be wide awake and very comfortable.

Submitted by Janet A Simons and Donald B Irwin.

144 TWENTY REASONS

This rapid-fire exercise stimulates thinking about the serious and not-so-serious reasons behind health-related behavior. This process can provide a lively introduction to any content area and is especially valuable with groups that are shy or reluctant to participate.

GOALS

To generate ideas on a specific topic.

To get group members involved.

GROUP SIZE

Unlimited.

TIME FRAME

5 minutes

PROCESS

1) The trainer chooses a topic related to the next content segment the group will consider (eg, smoking, nutrition habits, self-care, stress management, etc).

2) The trainer announces the topic to the group and explains the process.

   ➤ One of the first steps to changing behavior is understanding why we do what we do. With that in mind, this group is going to come up with 20 reasons why people behave the way they do. Specifically, why do people overeat?

   ☞ *Substitute the topic of your choice.*

   Suggestions: Why DO people smoke? Drink alcohol? Feel stressed? Get sick? Stay healthy? Exercise? Enjoy life?

   Why DON'T people exercise? Eat fish? Seek medical advice? Get sick? Reduce their salt intake? Meditate? Stop smoking?

   ➤ The goal is to accumulate a lot of reasons, both serious and not-so-serious.

   ➤ Each person should try to come up with a reason that hasn't previously been mentioned.

3) The trainer calls on each person in turn to give some sort of reason for the behavior.

☞ *Try to get everyone to participate. Encourage outlandish answers rather than no answers at all. Translate every comment (even "I don't know") into a reason (eg, lack of information, disinterest, confusion, etc).*

With a very large group, solicit at least 20 reasons from 20 different people. In a small group, keep going around until you have generated at least 20 reasons.

4) When the energy of the group starts to flag, the trainer summarizes the key serious and humorous points and uses this data to introduce the next content segment.

VARIATIONS

■ This same process with a different question makes an effective closing exercise. Ask participants to suggest 20 reasons why people should take this course. This affirmation helps people articulate the significance of what they have learned and provides valuable feedback for the trainer!

TRAINER'S NOTES

TRAINER'S NOTES

Resources

GUIDE TO THE RESOURCES SECTION

This resources section is intended to provide assistance for planning and preparation as you develop and expand your wellness training and health promotion consulting in various settings.

TIPS FOR TRAINERS p. 136

Suggestions for using audio-video materials in presentations, courses, and workshops.

EDITORS' CHOICE p. 138

Recommendations from the editors on their favorite exercises from **Wellness 4** and hints for on-the-job wellness training.

WINNING COMBINATIONS p. 142

Outlines for sessions of varying length using exercises from **Wellness 4** in combination. Plus notes on natural companion processes from other**Structured Exercises** volumes.

ANNOTATED INDEXES to Wellness 4 p. 144

Guides to specific content segments and group activities incorporated in exercises from **Wellness 4**, identified by page reference, time frame, brief description, and comments on use.

CONTRIBUTORS/EDITORS p. 150

Data on trainers who have shared their best process ideas in this volume. All are highly skilled educators and most provide in-house training, consultation, or workshops that may be valuable to you in planning comprehensive wellness programs. Many contributors are also established authors of well-respected materials on stress, wellness, and training issues.

WHOLE PERSON PUBLICATIONS p. 155

Descriptions of trainer-tested audio, video, and print resources available from the stress and wellness specialists.

TIPS FOR TRAINERS

Designing Presentations and Workshops Using
Structured Exercises in Wellness Promotion Volume 4

All of the exercises in this and other volumes of the **Structured Exercises** series are based on the model of experiential learning—creating opportunities for participants to interact with the concepts and each other in meaningful ways. The lecture method is replaced with succinct chalktalks and facilitative questions that guide people to discover their own answers. The "authority" of the trainer is transformed into the "authority" of the individual's inner wisdom.

Within this overarching educational framework, there is plenty of latitude for using all types of resources from guest experts to overheads to hypercard stacks and interactive video. Different media formats can be extremely valuable adjuncts to your training, as long as you don't let technology interfere with the goal of experiential learning. As a trainer, you are not presenting a paper at a conference. You are engaging an audience in an educational process. There is nothing more deadly than the "professional" presentation featuring one text-filled blue slide after another. When you turn out the lights, the audience often tunes out—unless you have prepared them to stay involved.

Exercise 117, **Health and Lifestyle**, p. 33 (60–90 min), is a good model for using audio- visual resources wisely, incorporating a short film as an information source and springboard for structured personal reflection and group interaction.

Audio-visual materials can be potent tools when they are well-integrated into your training strategy. Here are a few tips for using media effectively in training setting.

- **Match media to specific educational goals**. Import the experts or bring the real world into the training setting with video. Use it to introduce, reinforce, or summarize your content presentation, or to demonstrate a skill such as relaxation or stretching or assertiveness.

- **Use A-V for variety**. As you try to appeal to the diverse learning styles of your audience, audio and visual resources effectively reach folks who learn best in those channels and provide a change of pace for everyone. A-V is a great way to inject some humor into your presentation, with cartoons on overheads or a Bill Cosby clip that illustrate a key point.

- **Technology can enhance your image**. In some settings you will want to incorporate A-V materials in your training just to raise your credibility. The medical establishment expects slides, so give them a few. But use them in a way that stimulates active involvement rather than passive participation. Corporate America may expect action-packed video or slick overheads. Nothing wrong with that—as long as you also invite your audience to connect what they see and hear with their own life situations. When a topic is controversial or difficult, it's sometimes wise to raise the issue through

©1994 Whole Person Press 210 W Michigan Duluth MN 55802   (800) 247-6789

media. If there is resistance from the audience, you can play the "good guy" and let the "outside expert" take the flack.

Whenever you use A-V resources, be sure to fit the medium to your message and integrate it completely into your process design.

- If a video is supposed to deliver key content for the session, give people some warm-up that will engage their curiosity. Give them a list of things to watch for or intriguing questions that may be answered in the film. Brainstorm with the group beforehand what they imagine might be included in a film on this topic.

- Stop a film in the middle and ask people to predict what will happen next. Or stop several times for written reflection (individuals) or discussion (pairs/small groups) of what participants have learned or how they identify with the issues raised. Or stop as appropriate during the film to practice a skill, apply a principle, discuss alternatives.

- At the end, review the content by soliciting comments from participants or presenting your own summary points.

- But don't stop there. Develop a worksheet and process tailored to the film and your audience. Help people apply what they have seen and heard to their own life situation. Use the **Health and Lifestyles** exercise, p. 33, as a model.

A savvy trainer will also exercise some caution in using A-V resources. Fore-warned is forearmed.

- Always preview media. Know what you're going to show. Check films for in(ex)clusive language, stereotypes, diversity, appropriateness to the setting/audience.

- Expect something will go wrong. Be prepared. Don't depend on media services at the site to have everything in order. Go early and check out the equipment. If you are supplying your own equipment, make sure you have extra bulbs, long extension cords, etc.

- Always have a backup plan in case your A-V malfunctions.

A-V resources from posters to relaxation music to video to computer graphics can be powerful tools for learning. But don't be a slave to media. Remember—you and your participants are the best source of wisdom.

©1994 Whole Person Press 210 W Michigan Duluth MN 55802   (800) 247-6789

EDITORS' CHOICE

Although all 36 exercises in this volume are practical, creative, and time-tested, we must admit that we use some more often than others. When people call us and ask for suggestions about which exercises to incorporate into their workshop designs, we typically recommend some of our favorites—processes that have worked over and over again with many audiences, readings and activities that are guaranteed to charm a group. We call these our FOUR****STAR choices.

Four****Star Exercise	Page	Comments (Timing)
113 Wheel of Fortune	p. 11	Tried and true process that helps mix up a group and surprise people into new insights. Substitute conversation starters that fit your group and agenda. (10–15 min)
114 Wellness Emblem	p. 14	Simple process to help people focus on health issues, wellness principles, and personal goals—while they get acquainted. (15–20 min)
116 Whole Person Potpourri	p. 23	This exercise was a big hit at the National Wellness Conference. Great creative process to cap a daylong workshop. Works best with a big group and plenty of time. Teachers love it! (75–90 min)
121 Take a Walk!	p. 52	Most workshops and presentations have too much theory, not enough practice; too much talking, not enough action. Use this exercise to put some action and practical application into your training without sacrificing creativity and fun. (45–60 min)
123 Self-Esteem Grid	p. 52	Self-esteem continues to be a hot topic in the training world. Krysta Kavanaugh's 50-item checklist provides a helpful introduction to this elusive aspect of well-being. (45–50 min)
127 Let's Play	p. 79	A light-hearted look at a serious wellness strategy. Michael Metz's play-full process is perfect for the stressed out—from secretaries to senior management. (40–45 min)

©1994 Whole Person Press 210 W Michigan Duluth MN 55802   (800) 247-6789

ESPECIALLY FOR THE WORKPLACE

Most of the exercises in this volume are "generic" wellness processes that can be easily adapted to a variety of settings. When you are asked to conduct on-site health promotion programs, you may want to select content or processes that are particularly applicable in the workplace. All of the exercises listed below should be appropriate in nearly any job setting.

Workplace Exercise	Page	Comments (Timing)
109C TP Tales	p. 4	Offbeat icebreaker that loosens up a group. Works especially well in medical settings. (2 min per person)
111 Hearts at Risk	p. 6	Don Ardell has developed an inviting process for introducing the issue of risk factors and general health concerns related to heart disease. (10–15 min)
117 Health and Lifestyle	p. 33	Although this film is somewhat dated, it's still valuable for its wide view of wellness issues. The Variations section has lots of suggestions for special emphasis programs you can tailor to fit your setting and the specific wellness issues of your training (eg, alcohol use, cardiovascular risks, stress management, self-care). (60–90 min)
121 Take a Walk	p. 52	Great kickoff for a workplace walking campaign. Models support and creativity as components of a successful exercise program. (45–60 min)
128 Job Motivators	p. 85	Use the **Wheel of Fortune** (p. 11) as a warm-up to this in depth examination of needs and motivations. Participants determine their personal priorities for job satisfaction and compare them to the current job setting. (40–45 min)
131 Discoveries	p. 100	Through use of an in-session insight journal, this process models a potent self-care tool—periodic reflection and goal-setting. Works best in a longer workshop or multi-session course. (20–30 min)

141 New Sick Leave Policy   This employee benefit spoof should bring
                        p. 125 down the house. (5 min)

144 Twenty Reasons   p. 133 To close your session, try a variation of
                                this exercise where the group brainstorms
                                twenty reasons why other employees
                                should take your course. Bask in the
                                responses and then use them in your next
                                marketing campaign. (5 min)

WINNING COMBINATIONS

Health and Lifestyle Mini-Workshops (60–90 min)

You can use the film **Health and Lifestyle**, Exercise 117 (p. 33, 60–90 min) centerpiece for a mini-workshop on various wellness topics. The film provides and excellent overview of wellness concepts and provides a nice introduction for special-emphasis presentation. Mix and match exercises from this and other volumes of the **Structured Exercises** series for thematic presentations on topics such as:

> Whole Person Wellness
> Wellness with a Stress Management/Relaxation Focus
> Habit Control: Nutrition, Smoking, Alcohol Use
> Cardiovascular Disease Prevention

See the outlines on pp. 36–37 for details. The chalktalk notes and process design of this exercise are excellent, with or without the film.

Health Risks and Lifestyle Choices Presentation (60–90 min)

Follow the process described in Exercise 117, **Health and Lifestyle**, (p. 33 60–90 min) to explore the issues of stress, lifestyle, and risk factors. Use the icebreaker **Hearts at Risk**, Exercise 111 (p. 6, 10–15 min), for introductions and a warm-up to the topic of risk factors for cardiovascular disease or **Wellness Emblem**, Exercise 114 (p. 14, 15–20 min), for a more generic wellness orientation.

Don't miss the suggestion (p. 34) to stop the film and practice Herbert Benson's **Relaxation Response**. For a more extended closure/planning segment, add Exercise 130, **Beat the Odds**, (p. 97 10–15 min) or **So What?** (Stress 4, 10–15 min).

Wellness Presentation Focus: Self-Esteem (1–2 hours)

Self-esteem is a key component of well-being, an essential ingredient for responsible self-care. Start with the icebreaker **Wellness Emblem**, Exercise 114 (p. 14, 15–20 min), or the self-care introduction **Decades**, Exercise 120 (p. 49, (15–20 min).

Once participants are tuned in to some of their personal wellness history, focus in on the issues of self-esteem, the checklists and process in Exercise 123, **Self-Esteem Grid**, (p. 62 45–50 min). If you want to extend the depth of your presentation by expanding on the issues of stress and self-esteem, use **The Fourth Source of Stress** (Stress 2, 45–60 min).

Include some esteem-building energizers at appropriate points in the workshop. **Megaphone** (Wellness 1), **Cheers** (Wellness 2), and **Get Off My Back** (Stress 1) would fit well.

Close with the affirming process, **Whisper Circle**, Exercise 134 (p. 111, 10–15 min). Don't forget to step in the circle yourself for some positive feedback.

Play for the Health of It Workshop (90 min–3 hours)

Use Exercise 127, **Let's Play**, (p. 79 40–45 min) to put together a wellness training module for **Type As** and other over-responsible folks like professional helpers, who are likely to turn wellness into work.

Supplement the exercise with as many playful, on-the-spot exercises as possible. There are some great ones in this volume (**135 12 Days of Wellness**, p. 113; **138 Clapdance**, p. 118; **140 Joke Around**, p. 123; **141 New Sick Leave Policy**, p. 125) as well as several in other Structured Exercises (**Humorous Interludes**, Stress 1; **Month of Fundays**, Stress 2; **The Garden**, Stress 2; **Groans and Moans**, Stress 3; **Red Rover**, Wellness 1; **Outrageous Episodes**, Wellness 3). If you have time for a longer workshop, add another creative content segment. **Whole Person Potpourri**, Exercise 116 (p. 23, 75–90 min), uses a playful approach to defining whole person well-being and developing innovative strategies to move toward that vision of health. Or launch the group on a playful exercise adventure with Exercise 121, **Take A Walk** (p. 52, 45–50 min).

Close with Exercise 133, **Work of Art** (p. 108 30 min) where participants create personal "pop art" sculptures symbolizing their enlightened understanding of wellness.

ANNOTATED INDEXES

Index to CHALKTALKS

©1994 Whole Person Press 210 W Michigan Duluth MN 55802   (800) 247-6789

Index to DEMONSTRATIONS

Index to PHYSICAL ENERGIZERS

Index to MENTAL ENERGIZERS

©1994 Whole Person Press 210 W Michigan Duluth MN 55802   (800) 247-6789

Index to RELAXATION ROUTINES

©1994 Whole Person Press 210 W Michigan Duluth MN 55802   (800) 247-6789

CONTRIBUTORS

Donald B Ardell, Director, Wellness Institute, University of Central Florida, Orlando FL 32816. 407/823-2453. Don is the author of the landmark book **High Level Wellness: An Alternative To Doctors, Drugs, and Disease** and ten other books, including **Die Healthy** and **Freedom, Self-Management, and the Wellness Orgasm** (with Grant Donovan). He also publishes the quarterly **Ardell Wellness Report**, of which there are now 33 editions in print. (for a sample copy send a SASE to Dr Ardell).

Glenn Q Bannerman, President of Bannerman Family Celebration Services, Inc., Box 399, Montreat NC 28757. 704/669-7323. Professor Emeritus of the Presbyterian School of Christian Education, Richmond VA. Glenn is a specialist in church recreation and outdoor education. He has conducted workshops throughout the US, as well as overseas in 12 foreign countries. His group experiences range from movement exercises and clog dancing to gaming, puppetry, crafts, and camping. He is co-author of **Guide for Recreation Leaders**, and author of five LP American Mountain Music and Dance records.

Martha Belknap, MA. 1170 Dixon Road, Gold Hill, Boulder CO 80302. 303/447-9642. Marti is an educational consultant with a specialty in creative relaxation and stress management skills. She has 30 years of teaching experience at all levels. Marti offers relaxation workshops and creativity courses through schools, universities, hospitals and businesses. She is the author of **Taming Your Dragons**, a book and cassette tape of creative relaxation activities for home and school.

Lucia Capacchione, MA, PhD. PO Box 1355, Cambria CA 93428. 310/281-7495 (w), 805/546-1424 (h). Lucia is an art therapist, seminar leader, and corporate consultant. She is the author of nine books, including **The Creative Journal** (with versions for adults, teens and children), **The Well-Being Journal, Lighten Up Your Body, Lighten Up Your Life**, and **The Picture of Health**. After healing herself from a collagen disease through creative journaling, Lucia has dedicated her professional life to researching right brain approaches to healing and empowering individuals and organizations with new vision and innovative healing alternatives. Her best-known books, **The Power of Your Other Hand** and **Recovery of Your Inner Child**, open new doors to self-health.

Larry Chapman, MPH. President, Corporate Health Designs, PO Box 55056, Seattle WA 98155. 206/364-3448. Larry is a consultant, trainer and conference speaker. He has extensive experience in wellness programs in the workplace setting where he specializes in corporate health management, wellness programming, and designing benefit and incentive programs.

Grant Christopher, MD. Bemidji Clinic, 12333 4th St NW, Bemidji MN 56601. 218/751-1280 (w). Grant is a board certified family physician who practices and promotes the philosophy of wellness personally and professionally in his medical practice and through the teaching of seminars on wellness.

Lyman Coleman, MDiv, PhD. Serendipity House, Box 1012, Littleton CO 80160. 303/798-1313. Founder and director of Serendipity Workshops, Lyman has spent the past 30 years training over 150,000 church leaders of all denominations in small group processes. Author of scores of books, including a small group discussion version of the Bible, Lyman's innovative approach combines Bible study, group building and values orientation with personal story telling.

Dan Davidson, DC. Director, Spinal Care and Wellness Center, 3531 Keagy Road, Salem VA 24153. 703/989-5477. Dan writes wellness songs including the four theme songs he composed as publicity chairman for the annual "Roanoke Valley: Alive and Well" wellness week. He is president of "Alive and Well Music" which provides wellness education through song.

Joel Goodman, EdD. Director, The HUMOR Project, 110 Spring Street, Saratoga Springs NY 12866. 518/587-8770. Joel is a popular speaker, consultant and seminar leader who has presented to over 500,000 corporate managers, health care leaders, educators, and other helping professionals throughout the U.S. and abroad. Author of 8 books, Joel publishes **Laughing Matters** magazine and HUMOResources mail order bookstore catalog, and sponsors the annual international conference on "The Positive Power of Humor and Creativity."

Donald Irwin, PhD. Instructor, Des Moines Area Community College, Ankeny IA 50521. 515/964-6568. In addition to his teaching responsibilities, Don conducts numerous stress management workshops for audiences from house-keepers to University Regents' staff. Co-author of the textbooks, **Psychology—The Search for Understanding** and **Developmental Psychology—Understanding One's Lifetime**, Don manages his own stress by practicing for the Iowa State Fair hog-calling contest, where he has earned a blue ribbon three years in a row!

Krysta Eryn Kavenaugh, MA, CSP. 955 Lake Drive, St Paul MN 55120. 800/829-8437 (w) 612/725-6763 (h). Krysta is a speaker, trainer, and consultant. Her mission is to take people "into the heart of wisdom." She speaks with style, substance, and spirit. She is also the managing editor of **Marriage** magazine. Her favorite keynote topic is "Romancing Yourself: Taking Care of You is Taking Care of Business." She also speaks on proactive support teams, turning adversity to our advantage, ecology, and customized business topics.

Julie Lusk, MEd. Lewis-Gale Clinic, 1802 Braeburn Dr, Salem VA 24153. 703/772-3736. Julie is the editor of **30 Scripts for Relaxation, Imagery, and Inner Healing** (volumes 1 and 2). She works as the director of the Health management Center at Lewis-Gale Clinic and is the founder of the Alive and Well Coalition in Roanoke VA. Author of **30 Scripts for Relaxation and Imagery**, Julie leads workshops worldwide on a variety of topics and develops wellness programs for businesses, colleges, and communities. She is a licensed professional counselor and has taught yoga since 1977.

©1994 Whole Person Press 210 W Michigan Duluth MN 55802   (800) 247-6789

Michael Metz, PhD. Program in Human Sexuality, Univ of Minnesota Medical School, Ste 183, 1300 South 2nd Street, Minneapolis MN 55414. 612/625-1500. Licensed Psychologist, Licensed Marriage and Family Therapist, and a Clinical Member of the AAMFT. Originator of the Play Workshop for Couples, Mike has been researching the role of mature play in relationship intimacy for nearly a decade. He is currently coordinator of the marital and sexual therapy program.

Pat Miller, 1211 N Basswood Ave, Duluth MN 55811. 218/722-9361. Pat runs her own consulting and teaching business, Pat Miller Training and Development. She teaches workshops, conducts on-site team building sessions, facilitates retreats, and mediates conflict in the workplace. Her areas of expertise include communication skills, conflict resolution, team development, self-esteem, and stress management.

Janet Simons, PhD. Permanent Adjunct Faculty member, University of Iowa School of Social Work—Des Moines Extension. 220 Avalon Rd, Des Moines IA, 50314. 515/222-1999. Jan, a psychologist in private practice with the Central Iowa Psychological Services, has collaborated with Dr Donald Irwin on the textbooks **Psychology—The Search for Understanding** and **Developmental Psychology—Understanding One's Lifetime**.

Sondra Smalley, MA. Licensed Psychologist. Clinical Faculty Member, Univ of Minnesota Medical School. 12701 Tealwood Place, Minneapolis MN 55356. 612/449-0525. Sondra is a full time organizational consultant in the areas of self-directed work teams and collaboration.

Larry Tobin, MA. Jade Mist Press, 2529 SE 64th, Portland OR 97026. Larry is a special educator, school psychologist, and national trainer on working with troubled children. He has authored **What Do You Do with a Child Like This?**, **62 Ways to Create Change in the Lives of Troubled Children**, and **Time Well Spent**, a year-long stress management planner.

John Travis, MD, MPH. 21489 Orr Springs Rd, Ukiah CA 95482. 707/937-2331. John is the founder of the first Wellness Center, author of **Wellness Inventory**, and co-author of **The Wellness Workbook: Small Changes You Can Use To Make a Big Difference**, **Wellness for Helping Professionals**, and **A Change of Heart: A Global Wellness Inventory**. His commitment is to providing safe spaces, conflict resolution skills, and the experiences of co-operation and partnership for helping professionals—replacing the authoritarian mindset of the illness-care industry and the culture at large.

Neil Young, PhD. 728 14th Ave, Seattle WA 98122. 206/323-6310. Neil specializes in psychology and the arts, literature, and spirituality. As part of his concern for the wider world, he works regularly with Mother Teresa in Calcutta. He is currently developing a book on emphatic education.

FUTURE CONTRIBUTORS

If you have developed an exciting, effective structured exercise you'd like to share with other trainers in the field of stress or wellness, please send it to us for consideration, using the following guidelines:

● Your entry should be written in a format similar to those in this volume.

● Contributors must either guarantee that the materials they submit are not previously copyrighted or provide a copyright release for inclusion in the Whole Person **Structured Exercises** series.

● When you have adapted the work of others, please acknowledge the original source of ideas or activities.

EDITORS

All exercises in this volume not specifically attributed to other contributors are the creative efforts of the editors, who have been designing, collecting, and experimenting with structured processes in their teaching, training and consultation work since the late 1960s.

Nancy Loving Tubesing, EdD, holds a masters degree in group counseling and a doctorate in counselor education. She served as editor of the *Society for Wholistic Medicine's* monograph series and articulated the principles of whole person health care in the monograph, **Philosophical Assumptions**. Faculty Associate and Product Development Coordinator at Whole Person Associates, Nancy is always busy compiling and testing teaching designs for future **Structured Exercises** volumes.

Donald A Tubesing, MDiv, PhD, designer of the classic **Stress Skills** seminar and author of the best-selling **Kicking Your Stress Habits**, has been a pioneer in the movement to reintegrate body, mind, and spirit in health care delivery. With his entrepreneurial spirit and background in theology, psychology, and education, Don brings the whole person perspective to his writing, speaking, and consultation in business and industry, government agencies, health care, and human service systems.

Nancy and Don have collaborated on many writing projects over the years, beginning with a small-group college orientation project in 1970 and including two self-help books on whole person wellness, **The Caring Question** (Minneapolis: Augsburg, 1983) and **Seeking Your Healthy Balance** (Duluth: Whole Person Press, 1991), and a score of unusual relaxation audiotapes.

The Tubesings have specialized in developing creative stress management programs and packages for client groups such as the national YMCA (8-session course, **The Y's Way to Stress Management**) and Aid Association for Lutherans (**The Stress Kit** multimedia resource for families).

Their most recent efforts have been directed toward combining the process-oriented approach of the **Structured Exercises** series with the power of video. The resulting three six-session interactive video courses, **WellAware**, **Manage It!**, and **Managing Job Stress**, include participant booklets with worksheets that stimulate personal reflection and application of principles to specific situations, as well as a step-by-step leader manual for guiding group interaction.

About Whole Person Associates

At Whole Person Associates, we're 100% committed to providing stress and wellness materials that involve participants and have a "whole person" focus—body, mind, spirit, and relationships.

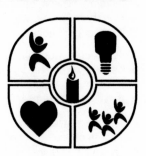

That's our mission and it's very important to us—but it doesn't tell the whole story. Behind the products in our catalog is a company full of people—and *that's* what really makes us who we are.

ABOUT THE OWNERS

Whole Person Associates was created by the vision of two people: Donald A. Tubesing, PhD, and Nancy Loving Tubesing, EdD. Since way back in 1970, Don and Nancy have been active in the stress management / wellness movement—consulting, leading seminars, writing, and publishing. Most of our early products were the result of their creativity and expertise.

Living proof that you can "stay evergreen," Don and Nancy remain the driving force behind the company and are still very active in developing new products that touch people's lives.

ABOUT THE COMPANY

Whole Person Associates was "born" in Duluth, Minnesota, and we remain committed to our lovely city on the shore of Lake Superior. All of our operations are here, which makes communication between departments much easier!

We've grown since our beginnings, but at a steady pace—we're interested in sustainable growth that allows us to keep our down-to-earth orientation—and put the same high quality into every product we offer.

ABOUT OUR EMPLOYEES

Speaking of down-to-earth, that's a requirement for each and every one of our employees. We're all product consultants, which means that anyone who answers the phone can probably answer your questions (if they can't, they'll find someone who can.)

We focus on helping you find the products that fit your needs. And we've found that the best way to do that is to hire friendly and resourceful people.

ABOUT OUR ASSOCIATES

Who are the "associates" in Whole Person Associates? They're the trainers, authors, musicians, and others who have developed much of the material you see on these pages. We're always on the lookout for high-quality products that reflect our "whole person" philosophy and fill a need for our customers.

Most of our products were developed by experts who are the tops in their fields, and we're very proud to be associated with them.

ABOUT OUR CUSTOMERS

Finally, we wouldn't have a reason to exist without you, our customers. We've met some of you, and we've talked to many more of you on the phone. We are always aware that without you, there would be no Whole Person Associates.

That's why we'd love to hear from you! Let us know what you think of our products—how you use them in your work, what additional products you'd like to see, and what shortcomings you've noted. Write us or call on our toll-free line. We're waiting for your call!

©1994 Whole Person Press 210 W Michigan Duluth MN 55802   (800) 247-6789